Intraductal Papillary Mucinous Neoplasm of the Pancreas

Masao Tanaka
Editor

Intraductal Papillary Mucinous Neoplasm of the Pancreas

Springer

Editor
Masao Tanaka
Department of Surgery and Oncology
Graduate School of Medical Sciences
Kyushu University
Fukuoka, Japan

ISBN 978-4-431-54471-5 ISBN 978-4-431-54472-2 (eBook)
DOI 10.1007/978-4-431-54472-2
Springer Tokyo Heidelberg New York Dordrecht London

Library of Congress Control Number: 2013950988

Printed on acid-free paper

Springer is part of Springer Science+Business Media (www.springer.com)

Preface

Approaches for the management of intraductal papillary mucinous neoplasms (IPMNs) of the pancreas have been evolving rather rapidly in recent years, owing to the increasing understanding of the natural history of those neoplasms based on observation and accumulation of histological data of surgically resected IPMNs. The strategy to manage main duct (MD)-IPMNs has not been greatly changed in terms of the indications for resection. However, we are taking a much more conservative approach nowadays to branch duct (BD)-IPMNs without high-risk stigmata of malignancy. This change from rather aggressive resection toward conservative surveillance is the principal alteration of the management strategy of BD-IPMNs adopted in the international consensus guidelines revised in 2012 after the Fukuoka meeting of the International Association of Pancreatology (IAP).

Although both of the IAP international consensus guidelines, issued in 2006 (Sendai) (see Tanaka et al. 2006 of Chap. 1) and revised in 2012 (Fukuoka) (see Tanaka et al. 2012 of Chap. 1), have contributed to increased awareness and more complete understanding of this entity, there are still many controversial or unknown features remaining to be clarified, in particular, with regard to the natural history and criteria for resection of BD-IPMNs. Since I found a carcinoma in situ (currently called high-grade dysplasia) concomitant with, yet distinct from, a benign small BD-IPMN for the first time in the world (see Tanaka et al. 1997 of Chap. 8), the association of IPMN and distinct pancreatic carcinoma recently has been drawing great attention. However, the precise incidence and pathophysiological significance remain to be elucidated. This book aims to review all aspects of our current knowledge about this fascinating entity. Because of the variety of physicians and scientists involved, I have directed the focus of the book to consider multiple disciplines, including internal medicine, radiology, surgery, and pathology. The content consists of four parts: pathophysiology, investigation, development of malignancy, and management of IPMNs, each of which comprises three to five chapters written by world experts of IPMN research institutions, including (in alphabetical order) the Aichi Cancer Center Hospital (Japan), the Johns Hopkins University (USA),

Kyushu University (Japan), the Massachusetts General Hospital (Harvard Medical School) (USA), the Mayo Clinic (USA), Seoul National University (Korea), the Teine Keijinkai Hospital (Japan), Tokyo Women's Medical University (Japan), and the University of Iowa (USA).

As the editor of this e-book, I sincerely hope that it be of great help to medical students, residents, fellows, and staff members of academic institutions as well as attending or practicing physicians in gastroenterology and gastrointestinal surgery.

Fukuoka, Japan Masao Tanaka

Contents

Part III Development of Malignancy

Part IV Management

Part I
Pathophysiology

Chapter 1
Macroscopic Morphological Classification and Its Significance

Masao Tanaka

Abstract Intraductal papillary mucinous neoplasms (IPMNs) are divided into three morphological types, i.e., branch duct type, main duct type, and mixed type, by radiological findings, most clearly by magnetic resonance cholangiopancreatography (MRCP). As in some previous analyses of resected IPMNs, histological classification of the IPMN types increases the frequency of mixed type of IPMN, because many branch duct (BD-) IPMNs show some degree of main duct involvement histologically. Correlation between the histologic and radiologic criteria is less than 80 %. The threshold of the main duct size for the diagnosis of a main duct (MD-) IPMN has been lowered from 10 to 5 mm in the revised Fukuoka international consensus guidelines. This lowered threshold recruits MD-IPMNs more sensitively without jeopardizing the specificity. MRCP is no doubt the best modality for the type classification by demonstrating the degree and extent of main duct dilation and the multiplicity of BD-IPMN. Multiple-type BD-IPMN accounts for 25–41 % of all BD-IPMNs. Whether the multiplicity actually multiplies the risk of malignant changes remains unknown. The guidelines recommend only segmental resection to remove the IPMNs at the highest oncological risk. The patients with any type of IPMN should be always informed with the possibility of total pancreatectomy according to the result of frozen section histology of the pancreatic stump.

Keywords Branch duct type • Intraductal papillary mucinous neoplasm • Main duct type • Malignant transformation • Mixed type • Pancreatic cancer

M. Tanaka (✉)
Department of Surgery and Oncology, Graduate School of Medical Sciences, Kyushu University, Fukuoka, Japan
e-mail: masaotan@med.kyushu-u.ac.jp

M. Tanaka (ed.), *Intraductal Papillary Mucinous Neoplasm of the Pancreas*,
DOI 10.1007/978-4-431-54472-2_1,

1.1 Definition

Intraductal papillary mucinous neoplasms (IPMNs) are divided into three morphological types, based on the distribution of dilated ducts, i.e., branch duct type, main duct type, and mixed type (Fig. 1.1). The mixed type is defined as generalized or segmental dilation of the main pancreatic duct along with dilation of one or more branches. The morphological classification should be determined by radiological findings obtained by imaging studies, most clearly by magnetic resonance cholangiopancreatography (MRCP), because the classification greatly affects the clinical management and the majority of the BD-IPMNs undergo conservative management without surgery (Tanaka et al. 2012). However, some analyses of resected IPMNs previously published based the type classification on histological findings (Salvia et al. 2004; Sohn et al. 2004). The histological classification of the IPMN types inevitably increases the frequency of mixed type of IPMN, because many BD-IPMNs show some degree of main duct involvement histologically. Correlation between the histologic and radiologic criteria is less than 80 % (Waters et al. 2008).

The threshold of the main duct size for the diagnosis of a MD-IPMN has been clearly determined as 5 mm in the revised international consensus guidelines (Fukuoka guidelines) (Tanaka et al. 2012). This threshold has been lowered from 10 mm, generally taken as the threshold, although not clearly defined, in the Sendai guidelines (Tanaka et al. 2006), to recruit MD-IPMNs more effectively. It has been

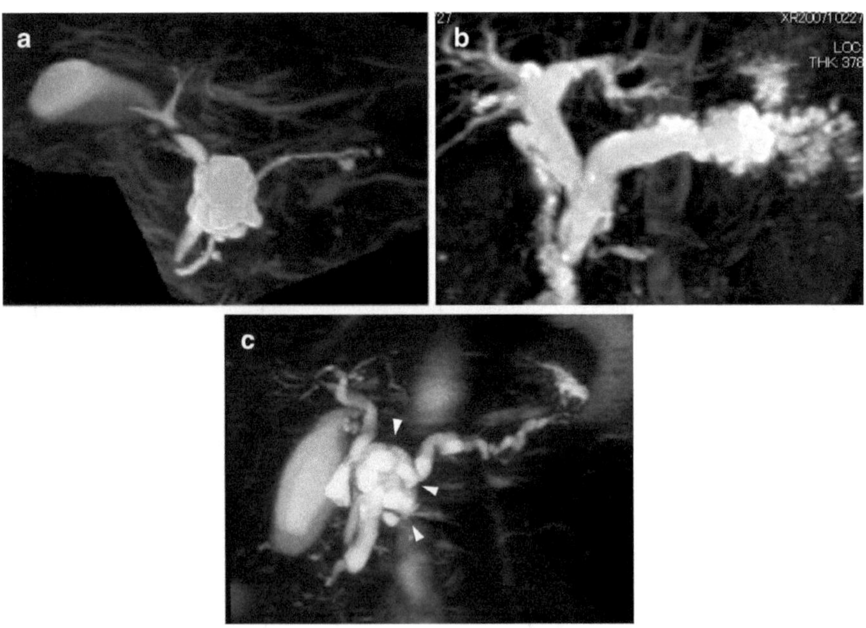

Fig. 1.1 MRCP images showing the classification of morphological type of IPMN. (**a**) Branch duct type. (**b**) Main duct type. (**c**) Mixed type

reported that this change increases the sensitivity of the diagnosis without jeopardizing the specificity (Schmidt et al. 2007; Hwang et al. 2012; Tanaka et al. 2012).

1.2 Method of Macroscopic Type Classification

The macroscopic classification of the IPMN types varies depending on the diagnostic radiologic methods to delineate IPMNs as well. Although almost all patients suspected as having IPMNs undergo ultrasonography, computed tomography (CT), and MRCP in Japan, this is not true in most other countries. For instance, of 214 patients with IPMN reported from Indianapolis in the United States, only 30 had both preoperative CT and MRCP (Waters et al. 2008). It is easily conceivable that this difference in utility of imaging studies may affect the accuracy of the type classification; however, this would not greatly influence the clinical management, because the presence of main duct dilation is relatively easy to detect somehow and the mixed type should be included in the main duct type in regard to the management. Anyway, MRCP is no doubt the best modality for the type classification by demonstrating the degree and extent of main duct dilation in main duct-type and mixed-type IPMNs (Fig. 1.2) and the multiplicity of BD-IPMN if any (Fig. 1.3).

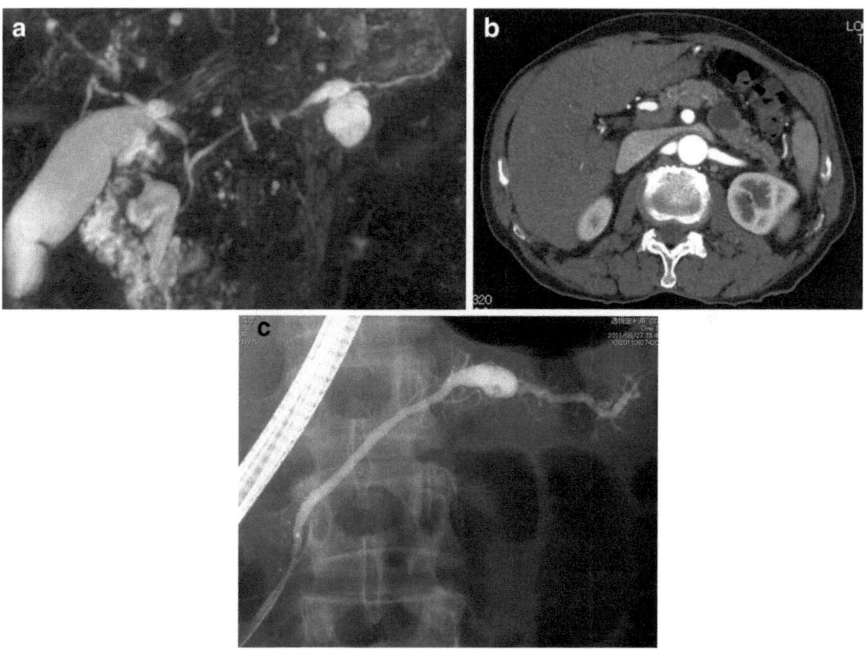

Fig. 1.2 Radiological images of mixed-type IPMN. (**a**) MRCP clearly delineating segmental dilation of the main pancreatic duct combined with a BD-IPMN. (**b**) CT scan demonstrating only multilocular dilated branches. (**c**) Endoscopic retrograde pancreatogram showing localized segmental dilation of the main pancreatic duct in the tail of the pancreas but no sufficient visualization of the dilated branch duct

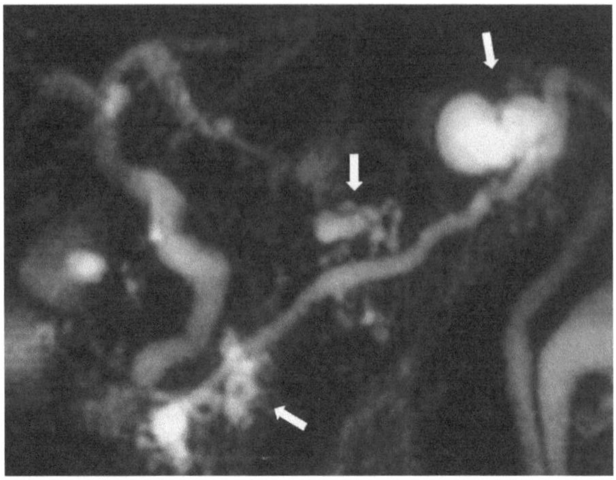

Fig. 1.3 MRCP showing multiple branch duct IPMNs

1.3 Relationship of Macroscopic Type Classification and Histological Subtypes

IPMN can be divided into four histological and morphological subtypes: an intestinal type, a gastric type, a pancreatobiliary type, and an oncocytic type. The histological subtypes were reported to be largely associated with macroscopic type classification of IPMNs. Of 283 patients reported by Furukawa et al. (2011), 137 had branch duct-type IPMNs, 102 main duct type, and 44 mixed type. Overall, the gastric type was the most common histological subtype (139 patients) and the intestinal type the next (101 patients), followed by far less common oncocytic type (24 patients) and pancreatobiliary type (19 patients). The gastric type was most frequent in BD-IPMNs (90 gastric, 28 intestinal, 12 oncocytic, seven pancreatobiliary), whereas the intestinal type was most common in MD-IPMNs (54 intestinal, 34 gastric, 19 pancreatobiliary, eight oncocytic).

When an IPMN becomes invasive carcinoma, most of the nonintestinal types (gastric, pancreatobiliary, and oncocytic type) progress into tubular carcinoma but the intestinal type into colloid carcinoma (Sadakari et al. 2010). The 5-year survival rate of patients with invasive IPMN derived from the nonintestinal type (0.0 %) was as poor as that of patients with conventional PDAC (19.9 %; $P=0.67$), while the patients with invasive IPMN derived from the intestinal type (66.7 %) had a more favorable prognosis than those with PDAC ($P<0.001$). Invasive IPMN arising from the nonintestinal type was characterized by positive lymphatic invasion and tubular invasive pattern. The same group of investigators confirmed their findings by analyzing the larger number of patients (179 resected IPMN) (Nakata et al. 2011). The prognosis was significantly better for patients with invasive IPMN derived from the intestinal type than for patients with invasive IPMN derived from the nonintestinal type ($P=0.013$). Tubular invasion ($P<0.001$) and lymphatic ($P=0.001$) or serosal ($P=0.021$) invasion were less frequently observed in intestinal-type IPMC than in nonintestinal-type IPMC. They concluded that invasive carcinoma derived from intestinal-type IPMN is more frequently associated with minimal invasion, colloid carcinoma, and less invasive behavior. Since the intestinal type is most commonly seen in the MD-IPMN, these characteristics also represent the clinicopathological features of the MD-IPMN. Although a multivariate analysis of 149 patients with resected IPMNs revealed that a dilated orifice of the duodenal papilla was also significantly associated with intestinal-type IPMN ($P<0.001$), this finding could not predict the malignant grade or distinguish the macroscopic types of IPMN (Aso et al. 2012).

Mino-Kenudson et al. (2011) also compared the study cohort comprising 61 patients with invasive IPMN and 570 patients with PDAC resected at Massachusetts General Hospital. The histology of invasive IPMN was tubular in 38 (62 %), colloid in 16 (26 %), and oncocytic in 7 (12 %). Compared with PDAC, invasive IPMNs were associated with a lower incidence of adverse pathological features and improved mortality by multivariate analysis (HR 0.58; 95 % CI 0.39–0.86). In subtype analysis, the favorable outcome remained only for colloid and oncocytic carcinomas, while tubular carcinoma of IPMN was associated with worse survival, not significantly different from that of PDAC (HR 0.85; 95 % CI 0.53–1.36). Specifically, this study could distinguish the intestinal and oncocytic types and mention the relationship to the macroscopic type classification. Colloid and oncocytic carcinomas arose only from the intestinal and oncocytic type IPMNs, respectively, and were mostly of the main duct type, whereas tubular carcinomas primarily originated in the gastric type, which was often associated with BD-IPMN (Mino-Kenudson et al. 2011).

1.4 Multiple-Type BD-IPMN (Fig. 1.3)

Twenty-five to forty-one percent of all BD-IPMNs are found in multiple sites of the pancreas (Fig. 1.3) (Schmidt et al. 2007; Waters et al. 2008; Rodriguez et al. 2007). Whether the multiplicity actually multiplies the risk of malignant changes remains unknown yet. Schmidt et al. (2007) reported that patients with symptomatic unifocal BD-IPMN are associated with a higher risk than those with symptomatic multifocal BD-IPMNs (18 % vs. 7 %). In theory, however, the number of BD-IPMNs reaching the malignant stigmata or worrisome features would affect the probability of malignancy in each patient. Nonetheless, the most recent guidelines recommend only segmental resection to remove the IPMNs at the highest oncological risk and perform surveillance of the remainders. Even in such cases, the patients should be always informed with the possibility of total pancreatectomy according to the result of frozen section histology of the pancreatic stump. IPMNs may be accompanied by multifocal PDACs (Mori et al. 2010). The guidelines also advocate that the threshold for total pancreatectomy should be lowered in those with a strong family history of pancreatic cancer in view of the increased prevalence of higher-grade dysplasia in such patients with IPMNs (Shi et al. 2009).

1.5 Type Classification Remaining Undetermined

There is a category not yet defined clearly. When IPMN involves the extreme periphery of the main pancreatic duct in the tail of the pancreas, the type classification is unclear (Fig. 1.4). Although their appearance looks like a BD-IPMN, whether this

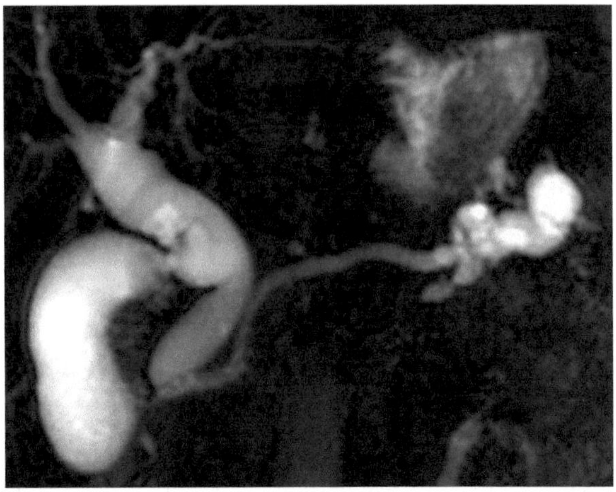

Fig. 1.4 MRCP depicting a solitary IPMN of undetermined type

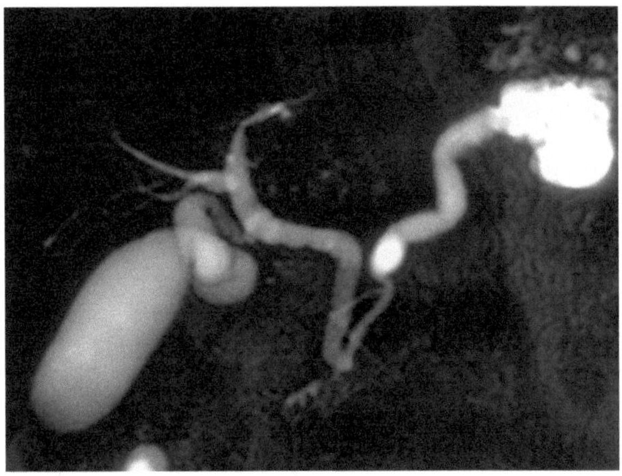

Fig. 1.5 MRCP demonstrating a "mixed-type" IPMN originating from an IPMN in the extreme periphery of the main pancreatic duct in the tail of the pancreas

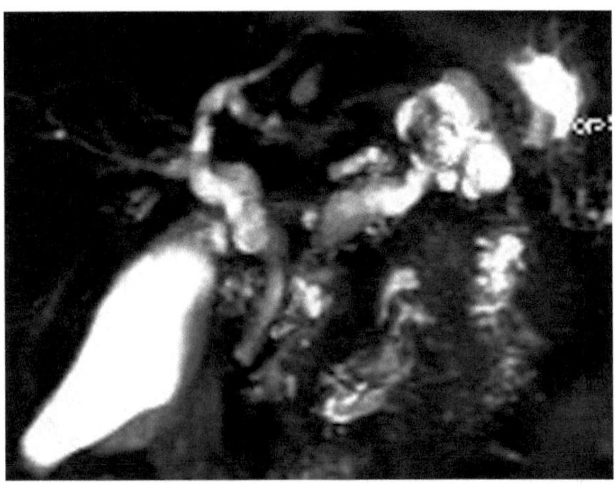

Fig. 1.6 MRCP taken 9 years after Fig. 1.3 in the same patient

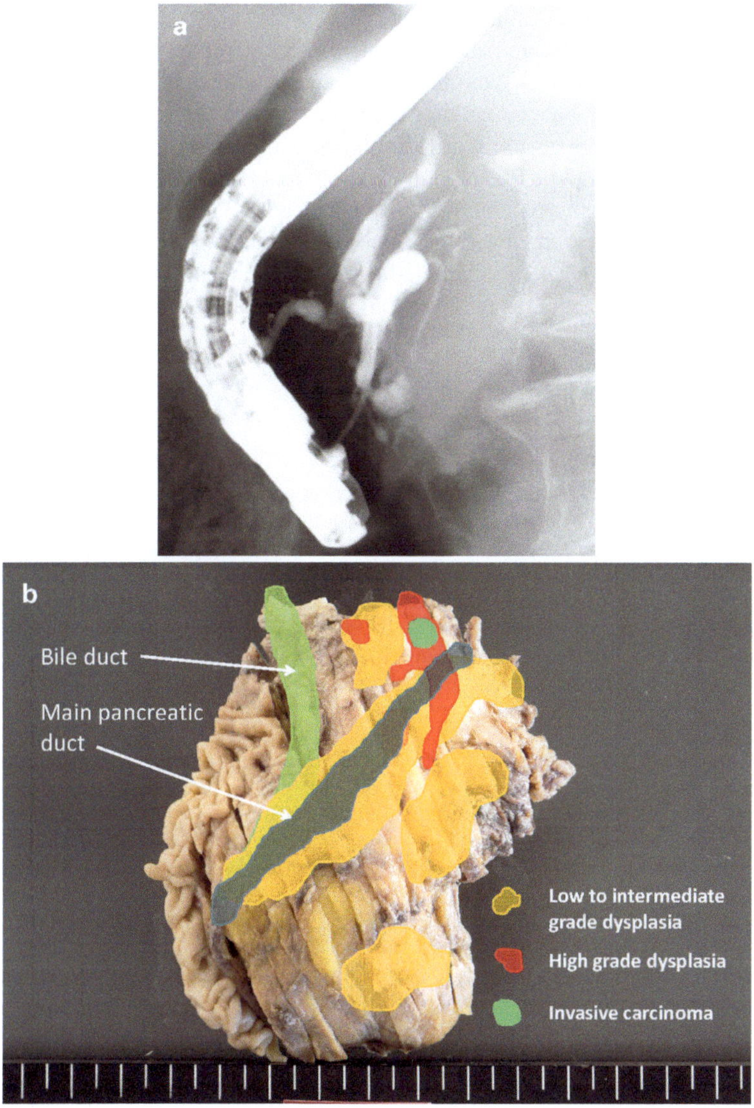

Fig. 1.7 Data obtained 5 years after distal pancreatectomy in the same patient as shown in Figs. 1.3 and 1.6. (**a**) ERCP showing generalized dilation of pancreatic ducts. Pancreatic juice cytology was positive for carcinoma. (**b**) Histological mapping of the specimen of total remnant pancreatectomy

type should be regarded as a branch duct type or a main duct type has not been clarified. When combined with main duct dilation, it appears to be a mixed type (Fig. 1.5). Figure 1.6 looks like a MD-IPMN, but this MRCP was taken 9 years after Fig. 1.3 in the same patient. The transition of ductal appearance in this patient suggests that the BD-IPMN at the extreme end of the duct in the tail of the pancreas can be the origin of the MD-IPMN actually observed 9 years later. This patient underwent distal pancreatectomy of "minimally invasive" IPMC proven by histology postoperatively. However, the main pancreatic duct in the preserved head of the pancreas became markedly dilated 5 years later, representing a MD-IPMN. Although there was no mural nodule, pancreatic juice cytology revealed carcinoma and the patient underwent total pancreatectomy of the remnant pancreas (Fig. 1.7). Histology disclosed extensive spread of IPMN in the main pancreatic duct and branches, one of which contained invasive carcinoma derived from with IPMN (Fig. 1.7b). More data in regard with clinical behavior, histological type and grade, and prognosis are needed to determine whether a branch duct-type-looking IPMN at the extreme end of the main pancreatic duct is really an early figure of a MD-IPMN.

References

Aso T, Ohtsuka T, Ideno N, et al. Diagnostic significance of a dilated orifice of the duodenal papilla in intraductal papillary mucinous neoplasm of the pancreas. Gastrointest Endosc. 2012;76:313–20.

Furukawa T, Hatori T, Fujita I, et al. Prognostic relevance of morphological types of intraductal papillary mucinous neoplasms of the pancreas. Gut. 2011;60:509–16.

Hwang DW, Jang JY, Lee SE, et al. Clinicopathologic analysis of surgically proven intraductal papillary mucinous neoplasms of the pancreas in SNUH: a 15-year experience at a single academic institution. Langenbecks Arch Surg. 2012;397:93–102.

Mino-Kenudson M, Fernández-del Castillo C, Baba Y, et al. Prognosis of invasive intraductal papillary mucinous neoplasm depends on histological and precursor epithelial subtypes. Gut. 2011;60:1712–20.

Mori Y, Ohtsuka T, Tsutsumi K, et al. Multifocal pancreatic ductal adenocarcinomas concomitant with intraductal papillary mucinous neoplasms of the pancreas detected by intraoperative pancreatic juice cytology. A case report. JOP. 2010;11:389–92.

Nakata K, Ohuchida K, Aishima S, et al. Invasive carcinoma derived from intestinal-type intraductal papillary mucinous neoplasm is associated with minimal invasion, colloid carcinoma, and less invasive behavior, leading to a better prognosis. Pancreas. 2011;40:581–7.

Rodriguez JR, Salvia R, Crippa S, et al. Branch-duct intraductal papillary mucinous neoplasms: observations in 145 patients who underwent resection. Gastroenterology. 2007;133:72–9.

Sadakari Y, Ohuchida K, Nakata K, et al. Invasive carcinoma derived from the nonintestinal type intraductal papillary mucinous neoplasm of the pancreas has a poorer prognosis than that derived from the intestinal type. Surgery. 2010;147:812–7.

Salvia R, Fernandez-del Castillo C, Bassi C, et al. Main duct intraductal papillary mucinous neoplasms of the pancreas: clinical predictors of malignancy and long term survival following resection. Ann Surg. 2004;239:678–87.

Schmidt CM, White PB, Waters JA, et al. Intraductal papillary mucinous neoplasms: predictors of malignant and invasive pathology. Ann Surg. 2007;246:644–51.

Shi C, Klein AP, Goggins M, et al. Increased prevalence of precursor lesions in familial pancreatic cancer patients. Clin Cancer Res. 2009;15:7737–43.

Sohn TA, Yeo CJ, Cameron JL, et al. Intraductal papillary mucinous neoplasms of the pancreas: an updated experience. Ann Surg. 2004;239:788–97.

Tanaka M, Chari S, Adsay V, et al. International consensus guidelines for management of intraductal papillary mucinous neoplasms and mucinous cystic neoplasms of the pancreas. Pancreatology. 2006;6:17–32.

Tanaka M, Fernández-del Castillo C, Adsay V, et al. International consensus guidelines 2012 for the management of IPMN and MCN of the pancreas. Pancreatology. 2012;12:183–97.

Waters JA, Schmidt CM, Pinchot JW, et al. CT vs MRCP: optimal classification of IPMN type and extent. J Gastrointest Surg. 2008;12:101–9.

Chapter 2
Natural History and Malignant Change of Main Duct IPMN

Klaus Sahora and Carlos Fernández-del Castillo

Abstract Among the exocrine tumors of the pancreas, intraductal papillary mucinous neoplasms (IPMNs) have gained increasing attention in the last decade. MD-IPMNs are predominantly (>50 %) composed of intestinal-type epithelium, producing thick mucus. In similarity to other epithelial neoplasms, MD-IPMN follows an "adenoma–carcinoma sequence" with progression into invasive cancer over the course of several years. On average, patients with malignant MD-IPMN are 4–6 years older than those with low- to moderate-grade dysplasia. There are no reliable predictors of malignancy for patients with MD-IPMN, although several studies have described clinical and radiologic features that are more common in MD-IPMN carcinoma. Like in ductal adenocarcinoma of the pancreas, jaundice and a recent onset or deterioration of diabetes mellitus are highly suspicious for malignancy. Significant effort has been made to understand the molecular pathogenesis of MD-IPMNs. Various molecular characteristics have been described in both MD-IPMN and BD-IPMN carcinoma, showing numerous parallels to conventional ductal carcinoma of the pancreas.

Keywords Cystic neoplasm • Intraductal papillary mucinous neoplasm • Pancreas • Surgery

---

K. Sahora
Department of Surgery, Medical University of Vienna, Waehringer Gvertel 18–20, Vienna 1010, Austria

C. Fernández-del Castillo (✉)
Wang Ambulatory Care Center, Massachusetts General Hospital, 15 Parkman Street, Boston, MA 02114, USA
e-mail: CFERNANDEZ@partners.org

M. Tanaka (ed.), *Intraductal Papillary Mucinous Neoplasm of the Pancreas*,
DOI 10.1007/978-4-431-54472-2_2, © Springer Japan 2014

2.1 Introduction

Among the exocrine tumors of the pancreas, intraductal papillary mucinous neoplasms (IPMNs) have gained increasing attention in the last decade. Due to the emerging number of people resected and observed with IPMN, numerous new insights have been made into its nature. Based on anatomic involvement of the pancreatic duct, IPMN of the pancreas are classified as main duct type (MD), side duct or branch duct (BD) type, and mixed or combined type. Radiologically, the characteristics of MD-IPMN are diffuse or segmental duct dilation in the absence of a stricture of the main pancreatic duct (Fig. 2.1), and pathologically it is characterized by intraductal growth of mucin-producing epithelial lining cells that have either a "flat" or papillary appearance.

It is without a doubt that IPMN of the main duct harbors a higher risk of malignancy compared to IPMN involving the branch ducts. In large surgical series, the rate of malignancy found in MD-IPMN is ~60 % (36–100 %) and the rate of invasive cancer, ~43 % (11–81 %) (Salvia et al. 2004; Suzuki et al. 2004; Crippa et al. 2010). We and others have shown that mixed or combined IPMN has epidemiologic features and a risk of malignancy that are very similar to IPMN that only affects the main pancreatic duct (Crippa et al. 2010).

Recently, important insights in the natural history of IPMN have been made by several authors, who have shown that the prognosis of invasive IPMN carcinoma is predominantly defined by its leading epithelial subtype (Ban et al. 2006; Mino-Kenudson et al. 2011; Maguchi et al. 2011). Currently, four epithelial subtypes of IPMN can be distinguished: an intestinal type, a pancreatobiliary type, an oncocytic type, and a gastric type (Furukawa et al. 2005b). The classification is based on the cytomorphological features of the papillae supported by the immunohistochemical features of mucin glycoproteins.

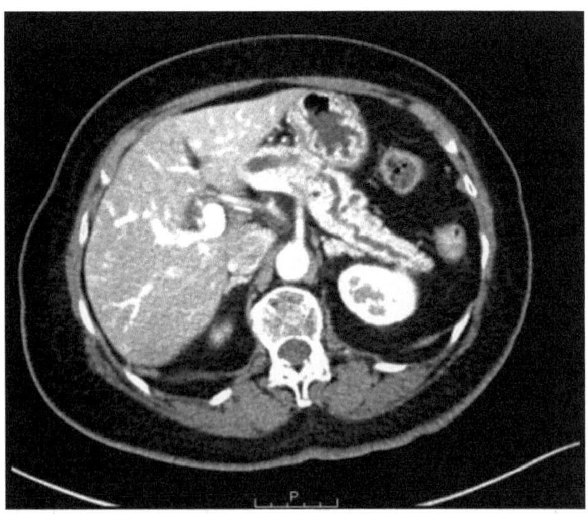

Fig. 2.1 Computed tomography of an MD-IPMN with diffuse dilation of the main duct

The *gastric-type* IPMN consists of cells mimicking gastric foveolae. This type usually shows low-grade atypia and rarely exhibits malignant transformation (Terris et al. 2002b). This subtype is of lower incidence in MD-IPMN and invasion is uncommon, but when it occurs, it is frequently of the more aggressive tubular carcinoma. *Intestinal-type* IPMN grows as intestinal villous neoplasms with tall columnar epithelial cells that usually demonstrate moderate- or high-grade atypia. This is the most frequent epithelial subtype expressed in main duct IPMNs. Malignant transformation is frequent in intestinal-type IPMN and invasive carcinomas arising from this type are more commonly of the colloid type and have a better prognosis (Adsay et al. 2001). The *pancreatobiliary-type* IPMN is less frequent than the intestinal type and shows complex papillary architecture. This group is often seen in an intimate mixture with less atypical gastric-type epithelium. Invasive carcinomas arising from this group are often the tubular type. The *oncocytic type* consists of cells with abundant, intensely eosinophilic cytoplasm and show complex thick papillae with intraepithelial lumina and severe high-grade atypia (Adsay et al. 1996).

MD-IPMNs are predominantly (>50 %) composed of intestinal-type epithelium, producing thick mucus, which characteristically produce a bulging major or minor papilla that can be viewed endoscopically. However, MD-IPMN can also be of the gastric subtype (~30 %), followed by the more rare oncocytic or pancreaticobiliary subtypes (Furukawa et al. 2011). As stated above, most invasive MD-IPMN carcinomas arising from the intestinal subtype are of the colloid and oncocytic subtype, and MD-IPMN carcinoma of these subtypes has a much better prognosis compared to conventional PDAC and tubular IPMN carcinoma (Mino-Kenudson et al. 2011).

2.2 Natural History in MD-IPMN

In similarity to other epithelial neoplasms, MD-IPMN follow an "adenoma–carcinoma sequence" with progression into invasive cancer over the course of several years (Salvia et al. 2010; Fernandez-Del Castillo and Adsay 2010). This hypothesis of an adenoma–carcinoma sequence has been supported by multiple studies that have shown a significant difference in the age of patients with benign and malignant MD-IPMN and is also supported by the fact that areas of low and moderate dysplasia are almost always seen in the vicinity of areas with invasive carcinoma. On average patients with malignant MD-IPMN are 4–6 years older than those with low- to moderate-grade dysplasia (Suzuki et al. 2004; Jang et al. 2005; Salvia et al. 2010).

According to data from Levy et al., the estimated occurrence of malignancy for MD-IPMN is estimated to be 58 % at 2 years and 63 % at 5 years after onset of symptoms (Levy et al. 2006). However, not every patient (only 58 %) in this study had histological confirmation of malignancy (high-grade dysplasia or invasive cancer). In a more recent analysis by Traverso et al., the progress to malignancy was much faster (50 % within 2 years) if pancreatitis-like symptoms were present (Traverso et al. 2012).

An ideal observational study of the natural history of MD-IPMN over time is missing and impractical to conduct; however, some insights have been gained from frail patients being treated conservatively for MD-IPMN. Although the overall number of observed individuals is very limited and final histological examination in those patients hardly exists, some authors claim the there might be a subset of main duct IPMN with a lower likelihood of malignancy.

Uehara et al. defined MD-IPMN with lower likelihood of malignancy as follows: a main pancreatic duct diameter of less than 10 mm, no visualized mural nodule, and a negative result of the cytological examination of pancreatic juice (Uehara et al. 2010). In that series of 20 observed low-risk MD-IPMN with a mean follow-up of 70 months, two patients progressed beyond low-risk criteria and underwent resection with the final diagnosis of invasive MD-IPMN carcinoma in one and carcinoma in situ in the second patient. The author concluded that selected MD-IPMN can be followed by close observation as long low-risk criteria are fulfilled. Another series published by Takuma et al. described the outcome of 20 patients with MD-IPMN who were conservatively followed because of high surgical risk due to major comorbidities (Takuma et al. 2011). After a median follow-up of 48 months, nine patients (45 %) died from their comorbidities, 3 (15 %) died of pancreatic cancer, and one patient was alive with documented conversion into pancreatic cancer. Of note, all patients who progressed into cancer demonstrated an increment of main pancreatic duct diameter. The revised international guidelines likewise defined a subset of MD-IPMN that may harbor a lower risk of malignancy: MPD dilation of 5–9 mm without other worrisome features (Tanaka et al. 2012). For this subset of MD-IPMNs, close observation is reasonable for surgically unfit patients.

2.3 Clinical and Radiological Changes Associated with Malignant Transformation of MD-IPMN

There are no reliable predictors of malignancy for patients with MD-IPMN, although several studies have described clinical and radiologic features that are more common in MD-IPMN carcinoma. Like in ductal adenocarcinoma of the pancreas, jaundice and a recent onset or deterioration of diabetes mellitus are highly suspicious for malignancy (Salvia et al. 2004). Other common symptoms include weight loss abdominal pain and steatorrhea. Radiologically, suspicious findings for malignant transformation in MD-IPMN are mural nodules or an associated mass, enhancement of the cyst wall, and a maximum main duct diameter of >10 mm (Manfredi et al. 2009; Sahani et al. 2006).

2.4 Molecular Changes in MD-IPMN

Significant effort has been made to understand the molecular pathogenesis of MD-IPMNs. Various molecular characteristics have been described in both MD-IPMN and BD-IPMN carcinoma, showing numerous parallels to conventional

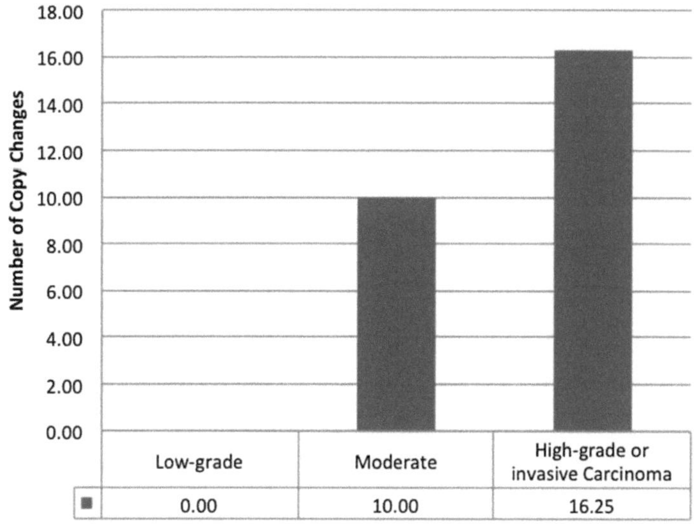

Fig. 2.2 Mean number of chromosomal gains/losses in IPMNs. The number of chromosomal gains and losses progresses as the degree of dysplasia advances in IPMN (Fritz et al. 2009)

ductal carcinoma of the pancreas. These include accumulation of K-ras mutations within the adenoma to carcinoma progression (Satoh et al. 1996; Kitago et al. 2004); loss of tumor suppressor pathways like *CDKN2A/p16/MTS1* due to mutation, deletion, or hypermethylation (Furukawa et al. 2005a; House et al. 2003); and abrogation of TP53 (Satoh et al. 1996). A study from the Massachusetts General Hospital, analyzing mainly combined and MD-IPMN, demonstrated that lesions with moderate- and high-grade dysplasia showed frequent chromosomal aberrations located on chromosome 5q, 6q, 10q, 11q, 13q, 18q, and 22q in a higher frequency than those found in low-grade IPMNs (Fritz et al. 2009) (Fig. 2.2). Other gene expression profiling studies of noninvasive vs. invasive IPMN have identified a panel of genes potentially associated with the invasive phenotype; i.e., Claudin 4, CXCR4, S100A4, and mesothelin were expressed at significantly high frequency in invasive IPMNs (Sato et al. 2004). Another small series has also identified several differentially expressed genes (caveolin1, glypican1, growth-arrest-specific 6 protein, cysteine-rich angiogenic inducer 61) throughout IPMN progression (Terris et al. 2002a). Although most of these molecular alterations are equally found in ductal adeno- and IPMN carcinoma of the pancreas, the incidence is generally lower in IPMN carcinoma (K-ras 60 % vs. 99 % (Soldini et al. 2003); TP53 8 % vs. 75 % (Goggins et al. 1999; Sessa et al. 1994).

A recently performed meta-analysis of genetic alterations in IPMN identified the expression of eight distinctive genetic markers in benign versus malignant IPMN: MUC1, MUC2, MUC5AC, kRas, p53, hTERT, Cox2, and Shh (Nissim et al. 2012). Pooled analysis of their data revealed expression of hTERT, Shh, and MUC1 to have the strongest association with malignant progression of IPMN.

References

Adsay NV, Adair CF, Heffess CS, Klimstra DS. Intraductal oncocytic papillary neoplasms of the pancreas. Am J Surg Pathol. 1996;20(8):980–94.

Adsay NV, Pierson C, Sarkar F, Abrams J, Weaver D, Conlon KC, et al. Colloid (mucinous non-cystic) carcinoma of the pancreas. Am J Surg Pathol. 2001;25(1):26–42.

Ban S, Naitoh Y, Mino-Kenudson M, Sakurai T, Kuroda M, Koyama I, et al. Intraductal papillary mucinous neoplasm (IPMN) of the pancreas: its histopathologic difference between 2 major types. Am J Surg Pathol. 2006;30(12):1561–9. doi:10.1097/01.pas.0000213305.98187.d4.

Crippa S, Fernandez-Del Castillo C, Salvia R, Finkelstein D, Bassi C, Dominguez I, et al. Mucin-producing neoplasms of the pancreas: an analysis of distinguishing clinical and epidemiologic characteristics. Clin Gastroenterol Hepatol. 2010;8(2):213–9. doi:10.1016/j.cgh.2009.10.001.

Fernandez-Del Castillo C, Adsay NV. Intraductal papillary mucinous neoplasms of the pancreas. Gastroenterology. 2010;139(3):708–13. doi:10.1053/j.gastro.2010.07.025.

Fritz S, Fernandez-Del Castillo C, Mino-Kenudson M, Crippa S, Deshpande V, Lauwers GY, et al. Global genomic analysis of intraductal papillary mucinous neoplasms of the pancreas reveals significant molecular differences compared to ductal adenocarcinoma. Ann Surg. 2009;249(3):440–7. doi:10.1097/SLA.0b013e31819a6e16.

Furukawa T, Fujisaki R, Yoshida Y, Kanai N, Sunamura M, Abe T, et al. Distinct progression pathways involving the dysfunction of DUSP6/MKP-3 in pancreatic intraepithelial neoplasia and intraductal papillary-mucinous neoplasms of the pancreas. Mod Pathol. 2005a;18(8):1034–42. doi:3800383 [pii] 10.1038/modpathol.3800383.

Furukawa T, Kloppel G, Volkan Adsay N, Albores-Saavedra J, Fukushima N, Horii A, et al. Classification of types of intraductal papillary-mucinous neoplasm of the pancreas: a consensus study. Virchows Arch. 2005b;447(5):794–9. doi:10.1007/s00428-005-0039-7.

Furukawa T, Hatori T, Fujita I, Yamamoto M, Kobayashi M, Ohike N, et al. Prognostic relevance of morphological types of intraductal papillary mucinous neoplasms of the pancreas. Gut. 2011;60(4):509–16. doi:10.1136/gut.2010.210567.

Goggins M, Kern SE, Offerhaus JA, Hruban RH. Progress in cancer genetics: lessons from pancreatic cancer. Ann Oncol. 1999;10 Suppl 4:4–8.

House MG, Guo M, Iacobuzio-Donahue C, Herman JG. Molecular progression of promoter methylation in intraductal papillary mucinous neoplasms (IPMN) of the pancreas. Carcinogenesis. 2003;24(2):193–8.

Jang JY, Kim SW, Ahn YJ, Yoon YS, Choi MG, Lee KU, et al. Multicenter analysis of clinicopathologic features of intraductal papillary mucinous tumor of the pancreas: is it possible to predict the malignancy before surgery? Ann Surg Oncol. 2005;12(2):124–32. doi:10.1245/ASO.2005.02.030.

Kitago M, Ueda M, Aiura K, Suzuki K, Hoshimoto S, Takahashi S, et al. Comparison of K-ras point mutation distributions in intraductal papillary-mucinous tumors and ductal adenocarcinoma of the pancreas. Int J Cancer. 2004;110(2):177–82. doi:10.1002/ijc.20084.

Levy P, Jouannaud V, O'Toole D, Couvelard A, Vullierme MP, Palazzo L, et al. Natural history of intraductal papillary mucinous tumors of the pancreas: actuarial risk of malignancy. Clin Gastroenterol Hepatol. 2006;4(4):460–8. doi:10.1016/j.cgh.2006.01.018.

Maguchi H, Tanno S, Mizuno N, Hanada K, Kobayashi G, Hatori T, et al. Natural history of branch duct intraductal papillary mucinous neoplasms of the pancreas: a multicenter study in Japan. Pancreas. 2011;40(3):364–70. doi:10.1097/MPA.0b013e31820a5975.

Manfredi R, Graziani R, Motton M, Mantovani W, Baltieri S, Tognolini A, et al. Main pancreatic duct intraductal papillary mucinous neoplasms: accuracy of MR imaging in differentiation between benign and malignant tumors compared with histopathologic analysis. Radiology. 2009;253(1):106–15. doi:10.1148/radiol.2531080604.

Mino-Kenudson M, Fernandez-Del Castillo C, Baba Y, Valsangkar NP, Liss AS, Hsu M, et al. Prognosis of invasive intraductal papillary mucinous neoplasm depends on histological and precursor epithelial subtypes. Gut. 2011;60(12):1712–20. doi:10.1136/gut.2010.232272.

Nissim S, Idos GE, Wu B. Genetic markers of malignant transformation in intraductal papillary mucinous neoplasm of the pancreas: a meta-analysis. Pancreas. 2012. doi:10.1097/MPA.0b013e3182580fb4.

Sahani DV, Kadavigere R, Blake M, Fernandez-Del Castillo C, Lauwers GY, Hahn PF. Intraductal papillary mucinous neoplasm of pancreas: multi-detector row CT with 2D curved reformations–correlation with MRCP. Radiology. 2006;238(2):560–9. doi:10.1148/radiol.2382041463.

Salvia R, Fernandez-Del Castillo C, Bassi C, Thayer SP, Falconi M, Mantovani W, et al. Main-duct intraductal papillary mucinous neoplasms of the pancreas: clinical predictors of malignancy and long-term survival following resection. Ann Surg. 2004;239(5):678–85. discussion 685–677.

Salvia R, Crippa S, Partelli S, Armatura G, Malleo G, Paini M, et al. Differences between main-duct and branch-duct intraductal papillary mucinous neoplasms of the pancreas. World J Gastrointest Surg. 2010;2(10):342–6. doi:10.4240/wjgs.v2.i10.342.

Sato N, Fukushima N, Maitra A, Iacobuzio-Donahue CA, van Heek NT, Cameron JL, et al. Gene expression profiling identifies genes associated with invasive intraductal papillary mucinous neoplasms of the pancreas. Am J Pathol. 2004;164(3):903–14. doi:S0002-9440(10)63178-1 [pii] 10.1016/S0002-9440(10)63178-1.

Satoh K, Shimosegawa T, Moriizumi S, Koizumi M, Toyota T. K-ras mutation and p53 protein accumulation in intraductal mucin-hypersecreting neoplasms of the pancreas. Pancreas. 1996;12(4):362–8.

Sessa F, Solcia E, Capella C, Bonato M, Scarpa A, Zamboni G, et al. Intraductal papillary-mucinous tumours represent a distinct group of pancreatic neoplasms: an investigation of tumour cell differentiation and K-ras, p53 and c-erbB-2 abnormalities in 26 patients. Virchows Arch. 1994;425(4):357–67.

Soldini D, Gugger M, Burckhardt E, Kappeler A, Laissue JA, Mazzucchelli L. Progressive genomic alterations in intraductal papillary mucinous tumours of the pancreas and morphologically similar lesions of the pancreatic ducts. J Pathol. 2003;199(4):453–61. doi:10.1002/path.1301.

Suzuki Y, Atomi Y, Sugiyama M, Isaji S, Inui K, Kimura W, et al. Cystic neoplasm of the pancreas: a Japanese multiinstitutional study of intraductal papillary mucinous tumor and mucinous cystic tumor. Pancreas. 2004;28(3):241–6.

Takuma K, Kamisawa T, Anjiki H, Egawa N, Kurata M, Honda G, et al. Predictors of malignancy and natural history of main-duct intraductal papillary mucinous neoplasms of the pancreas. Pancreas. 2011;40(3):371–5. doi:10.1097/MPA.0b013e3182056a83.

Tanaka M, Fernandez-Del Castillo C, Adsay V, Chari S, Falconi M, Jang J-Y, et al. International consensus guidelines 2012 for the management of IPMN and MCN of the pancreas. Pancreatology. 2012;12(3):183–97. doi:10.1016/j.pan.2012.04.004.

Terris B, Blaveri E, Crnogorac-Jurcevic T, Jones M, Missiaglia E, Ruszniewski P, et al. Characterization of gene expression profiles in intraductal papillary-mucinous tumors of the pancreas. Am J Pathol. 2002a;160(5):1745–54. doi:S0002-9440(10)61121-2 [pii] 10.1016/S0002-9440(10)61121-2.

Terris B, Dubois S, Buisine MP, Sauvanet A, Ruszniewski P, Aubert JP, et al. Mucin gene expression in intraductal papillary-mucinous pancreatic tumours and related lesions. J Pathol. 2002b;197(5):632–7. doi:10.1002/path.1146.

Traverso LW, Moriya T, Hashimoto Y. Intraductal papillary mucinous neoplasms of the pancreas: making a disposition using the natural history. Curr Gastroenterol Rep. 2012;14(2):106–11. doi:10.1007/s11894-012-0239-7.

Uehara H, Ishikawa O, Ikezawa K, Kawada N, Inoue T, Takakura R, et al. A natural course of main duct intraductal papillary mucinous neoplasm of the pancreas with lower likelihood of malignancy. Pancreas. 2010;39(5):653–7. doi:10.1097/MPA.0b013e3181c81b52.

Chapter 3
Natural History and Malignant Transformation of Branch Duct IPMN

Hiroyuki Maguchi and Satoshi Tanno

Abstract The number of reports published on the follow-up data of patients with BD-IPMN has been increasing. Accumulating evidence from independent 12 studies revealed that the mean frequency of morphological changes of BD-IPMN, such as increased cyst size, increased MPD diameter, and/or appearance or enlargement of MNs, was 27.4 % (range, 14.9–61.8 %) of 1,293 followed-up patients (follow-up period, 2.6–8.1 years). Surgical resection was carried out in 9.9 % (range, 0–22.2 %) of all cases. Among the resected cases, 27.3 % were diagnosed histologically as malignant. During the follow-up period, malignant transformation was observed in only 2.7 %. BD-IPMNs without MNs have a low risk for malignant transformation regardless of cyst size at the initial diagnosis. Malignant transformation is associated with signs of progression especially appearance or enlargement of MNs and/or an increase in the MPD diameter. On the other hand, PDAC develops independently in the pancreas distinct from BD-IPMN. The mean frequency of PDAC occurrence was 2.8 % (range, 1.4–8.0 %) of all cases during the follow-up.

In conclusion, careful attention should be paid to the occurrence of PDAC in the entire pancreas in addition to progression of BD-IPMN when performing follow-up examinations in patients with BD-IPMN.

Keywords BD-IPMN • BD-IPMNs without MNs • Follow-up • Guideline 2012 • Malignant transformation • MNs • Morphological changes • MPD diameter • Natural history • Pancreatic ductal adenocarcinoma (PDAC) • PDAC concomitant with IPMN • Progression

H. Maguchi (✉)
Center for Gastroenterology, Teine-Keijinkai Hospital, Sapporo, Japan
e-mail: maguchi@tb3.so-net.ne.jp

S. Tanno
Department of Gastroenterology, Sapporo Gastroenterology Center General Hospital, Sapporo, Japan

M. Tanaka (ed.), *Intraductal Papillary Mucinous Neoplasm of the Pancreas*,
DOI 10.1007/978-4-431-54472-2_3,

3.1 Introductory Remarks

IPMNs can be classified into three types, i.e., main duct IPMN (MD-IPMN), branch duct IPMN (BD-IPMN), and mixed type, based on imaging study and/or the histology in the revised guidelines (Tanaka et al. 2012). The frequency of malignant BD-IPMN such as IPMN with high-grade dysplasia or noninvasive cancer and IPMN with an associated invasive cancer is lower than that of MD-IPMN and mixed type (Tanaka et al. 2012). Patients with BD-IPMN who do not have any sign of malignancy may be managed conservatively.

Although the natural history of BD-IPMN is not well established, there have been an increasing number of reports published on the follow-up data in patients with BD-IPMN.

3.2 Morphological Change of BD-IPMN During the Follow-Up Period

The published reports on the follow-up of BD-IPMN were summarized in Table 3.1 (Kobayashi et al. 2005; Lee et al. 2007; Rautou et al. 2008; Tanno et al. 2008; Guarise et al. 2008; Sawai et al. 2010; Uehara et al. 2011; Maguchi et al. 2011; Arlix et al. 2012; Bae et al. 2012; Ohno et al. 2012; Khannoussi et al. 2012). Total number of cases was 1,293. The range of mean initial cyst size and main pancreatic duct (MPD) diameter was 15–28 mm and 2.4–3.8 mm, respectively. Almost all

Table 3.1 Morphological changes of BD-IPMN during follow-up

		Initial imaging findings				
Author (year)	Number of cases	Cyst size (mm)	MPD (mm)	MN (absent/ present)	Progression (%)	Follow-up period (year)
Kobayashi et al. (2005)	47	28	–	10/37	7 (14.9)	3.5
Lee et al. (2007)	45	28	–	–	10 (22.2)	3.5
Rautou et al. (2008)	121	15	–	–	33 (27.3)	2.8
Tanno et al. (2008)	82	20	3	0/82	13 (15.9)	8.1
Guarise et al. (2008)	52	17	2.8	11/41	11 (21.2)	2.6
Sawai et al. (2010)	103	18	3	–	29 (28.2)	4.9
Uehara et al. (2011)	100	21	3.8	5/95	28 (28.0)	5.1
Maguchi et al. (2011)	349	19	3	0/349	62 (17.8)	3.7
Arlix et al. (2012)	47	15	2.4	0/47	18 (38.3)	6.4
Bae et al. (2012)	152	22	–	–	94 (61.8)	2.6
Ohno et al. (2012)	142	22	2.5	61/81	35 (24.6)	3.5
Khannoussi et al. (2012)	53	–	–	–	15 (28.3)	7.0
Total	1,293				355 (27.4)	

MPD main pancreatic duct, *MN* mural nodule

cases were suspected to have a low risk of malignancy. The mean follow-up period ranged from 2.6 to 8.1 years.

Among these, the mean frequency of morphological changes on the imaging findings, such as increased cyst size, increased MPD diameter, and/or appearance or enlargement of mural nodules (MNs), was 27.4 % (335/1,293) (range, 14.9–61.8 %) of all cases during the follow-up period.

There are several reasons for varying the range in frequency. The most obvious reason may be the different definition of the progression of BD-IPMN especially in cyst size. Some authors have defined cyst size changes of 5–10 mm or greater as progression (Rautou et al. 2008; Maguchi et al. 2011) because of the difficulty in the accurate measuring of a grape-like dilated cyst. However, Bae et al. (2012) reported that 94 (61.8 %) of 152 patients showed an increase in cyst size, and the mean incremental rate of cyst size growth was 0.0038 cm/month. Arlix et al. (2012) also reported that 18 (38.3 %) of 47 patients showed an increased cyst size, and the mean enlarged size was less than 3 mm.

Other reasons include differences in the patient characteristics at the initial diagnosis, the difference of imaging modalities in each institution, and the difference of the follow-up periods.

3.3 Malignant Transformation of BD-IPMN During the Follow-Up

The number of resected cases with BD-IPMN during the follow-up was shown in Table 3.2 (Kobayashi et al. 2005; Lee et al. 2007; Rautou et al. 2008; Tanno et al. 2008; Guarise et al. 2008; Sawai et al. 2010; Uehara et al. 2011; Maguchi et al. 2011; Arlix et al. 2012; Bae et al. 2012; Ohno et al. 2012; Khannoussi et al. 2012). The mean frequency of resected cases was 9.9 % (128/1,293) (range, 0–22.2 %) of all cases. Of 128 BD-IPMNs, 35 (27.3 %) cases were diagnosed histologically as malignant (noninvasive 25 and invasive 10). Therefore, the frequency of malignant transformation was only 2.7 % (35/1,293) in total during the follow-up period, whereas the remaining patients without surgical resection may have a risk of malignant transformation in the future.

Thirty-two (91.4 %) of 35 patients with malignant BD-IPMNs exhibited obvious signs of progression such as increased cyst size, increased MPD diameter, and/or appearance or enlargement of MNs. Three (8.5 %) malignant cases having no change of cyst size or MPD diameter showed an appearance of a solid mass at the periphery of the cyst during the follow-up (Kobayashi et al. 2005).

In addition, a multicenter study in Japan (Maguchi et al. 2011) reported that all nine malignant BD-IPMN cases exhibited progression, although all seven patients with benign BD-IPMN had no progression during the follow-up period.

These findings support the notion that malignancy is associated with signs of progression.

Table 3.2 Resected cases of BD-IPMN during follow-up

Author (year)	Number of resected cases (%)	Malignancy of resected cases		Histological findings of malignancy	
		Progression	No change	Noninvasive	Invasive
Kobayashi et al. (2005)	6 (12.8)	0/3	3[a]/3		3[a]
Lee et al. (2007)	10 (22.2)	2/10		1	1
Rautou et al. (2008)	8 (6.7)	4/8		4	
Tanno et al. (2008)	7 (8.5)	1/7		1	
Guarise et al. (2008)	0				
Sawai et al. (2010)	11 (10.7)	3/8	0/3	2	1
Uehara et al. (2011)	1 (1)	1/1		1	
Maguchi et al. (2011)	29 (8.3)	9/22	0/7	8	1
Arlix et al. (2012)	5 (10.2)	0/5			
Bae et al. (2012)	18 (11.8)	3/18		2	1
Ohno et al. (2012)	30 (21.1)	9/30		6	3
Khannoussi et al. (2012)	3 (5.7)	0/3			
Total	128 (9.9)	32/115	3[a]/13	25	10

[a]No change of cyst size and MPD diameter except the appearance of a solid mass at the periphery of the cyst

Table 3.3 Progression and malignancy of BD-IPMN without MN during follow-up

Author (year)	Number of cases	Progression (%)	Malignant (%)	IPMN with an associated invasive carcinoma (%)	Follow-up period (year)
Kobayashi et al. (2005)	29	0	0	0	3.5
Tanno et al. (2008)	82	13 (15.9)	1 (1.2)	0	8.1
Guarise et al. (2008)	41	4 (9.7)	0	0	2.6
Uehara et al. (2011)	95	7[a] (7.4)	2 (2.1)	1(1.1)	5.1
Maguchi et al. (2011)	349	62 (17.8)	9 (2.6)	1 (0.3)	3.7
Arlix et al. (2012)	47	18 (36.7)	0	0	6.4
Total	643	104 (16.2)	12(1.9)	2(0.3)	

[a]Appearance of MN alone

3.4 Progression and Malignancy of BD-IPMN Without MNs

The presence of MNs has been reported to be strongly suggestive of malignancy. Table 3.3 shows the follow-up data of BD-IPMN patients who had no MNs at the initial diagnosis (Kobayashi et al. 2005; Tanno et al. 2008; Guarise et al. 2008; Uehara et al. 2011; Maguchi et al. 2011; Arlix et al. 2012). The mean frequency of progression was 16.2 % (104/643) of all cases during the follow-up period. Twelve (1.9 %) cases were found to be malignant by histological examination, and only two (0.3 %) cases were IPMN with an associated invasive cancer.

These findings suggest that BD-IPMNs without MNs have a low risk of progression and malignant transformation. They are suitable for management without surgery and do not need short interval surveillance.

Table 3.4 Initial cyst size in relation to progression and malignancy

Author (year)	Number of cases (%)	Progression (%)	Malignant (%)
Tanno et al. (2008)			
<3 cm	72 (87.8)	10 (13.9)	1 (1.4)
≧3 cm	10 (12.2)	3 (30.0)	0
Maguchi et al. (2011)			
<3 cm	287 (82.2)	49 (17.1)	6 (2.1)
≧3 cm	62 (17.8)	13 (21.0)	3 (4.8)

3.5 Cyst Size in Relation to Progression and Malignancy

Cyst size >3 cm was previously thought to be one of the predictors of malignancy. Therefore, a BD-IPMN >3 cm was included in the consensus criteria for resection in the first guidelines (Tanaka et al. 2006).

Several studies have validated the safety of this guideline for surgical treatment of BD-IPMN >3 cm and revealed that the specificity is quite low (Rodriguez et al. 2007; Tang et al. 2008; Pelaez-Luna et al. 2007). These reports suggest that a BD-IPMN size of >3 cm is a weaker indicator of malignancy than the presence of MNs (Tanaka et al. 2012).

There was few number of long-term follow-up data in patients with BD-IPMN >3 cm. Table 3.4 shows the initial cyst size in relation to progress and malignancy during the follow-up (Tanno et al. 2008; Maguchi et al. 2011). Two studies demonstrated that there was no significant difference in the frequency of progression and malignancy in the resected cases between initial cyst size of less than 3 and 3 cm or greater.

With accordance to this, the revised guideline 2012 recommends that the indication for resection is more conservative (Tanaka et al. 2012). BD-IPMN >3 cm without any signs of further risk stratification can be observed without immediate resection.

3.6 Predictive Sign of Malignancy During Follow-Up

Although malignancy is associated with sign of progression of BD-IPMN during follow-up, adequate predictive signs of malignancy have not been defined. Many investigators proposed signs of malignancy as the appearance or the enlargement of MNs and/or an increase in MPD diameter (Lee et al. 2007; Tanno et al. 2008; Sawai et al. 2010; Uehara et al. 2011; Maguchi et al. 2011; Ohno et al. 2012). It is still controversial whether an increase in cyst size alone is an adequate predictive sign of malignancy (Rautou et al. 2008; Bae et al. 2012; Kang et al. 2011) or not (Lee et al. 2007; Tanno et al. 2008; Sawai et al. 2010; Uehara et al. 2011; Maguchi et al. 2011; Ohno et al. 2012).

3.7 Pancreatic Ductal Adenocarcinoma in Patients with BD-IPMN

Pancreatic ductal adenocarcinoma (PDAC) may develop independently in the pancreas separately from IPMNs, especially in BD-IPMN (Tanaka et al. 2012; Yamaguchi et al. 2002). The frequency of PDAC concomitant with IPMN was 4.1–9.3 % in the resected case studies (Yamaguchi et al. 2002; Ingakul et al. 2010; Kanno et al. 2010; Tanno et al. 2010a; Yamaguchi et al. 2011).

During the last several years, an increasing number of reports for the occurrence of PDAC in follow-up patients with IPMN have been published (Sawai et al. 2010; Uehara et al. 2011; Maguchi et al. 2011; Tada et al. 2006; Uehara et al. 2008; Tanno et al. 2010b; Ikeuchi et al. 2010) (Table 3.5). The mean frequency of occurrence of PDAC concomitant with IPMN was 2.8 % (range, 1.4–8.0 %) during follow-up. It is noted that the frequency (2.8 %, 30/1,085) was similar to the frequency of malignant transformation of BD-IPMN (2.7 %, 35/1,293) during the follow-up.

These findings suggest that BD-IPMN may be an indicator for a precancerous state of the pancreas and that PDAC may have not infrequently occurred in the pancreas distinct from BD-IPMN.

The long-term prognosis of the patients with BD-IPMN is still unclear. However, a multicenter study in Japan (Maguchi et al. 2011) described that the patients with PDAC distinct from BD-IPMN had a poor prognosis, whereas patients with malignant BD-IPMNs, including noninvasive and invasive carcinomas, had a relatively better prognosis after surgical treatment.

In conclusion, special attention should be paid to the occurrence of PDAC in the entire pancreas when performing follow-up examinations in patients with BD-IPMN including postoperative status, and shorter interval surveillance is required.

Table 3.5 Occurrence of PDAC in patients with BD-IPMN during follow-up

Author (year)	Number of cases	Number of PDAC concomitant with IPMN (%)	Follow-up period (year)
Tada et al. (2006)	197[a]	5 (2.6)	3.8
Uehara et al. (2008)	60	5 (8.0)	7.3
Tanno et al. (2010b)	89	4 (4.5)	5.3
Ikeuchi et al. (2010)	145	5 (3.4)	4.6
Sawai et al. (2010)	103	2 (1.9)	4.9
Maguchi et al. (2011)	349	7 (2.0)	3.7
Ohno et al. (2012)	142	2 (1.4)	3.5
Total	1,085	30 (2.8)	

[a]Included pancreatic cyst

References

Arlix A, Bournet B, Otal P, et al. Long-term clinical and imaging follow-up of nonoperated branch duct form of intraductal papillary mucinous neoplasms of the pancreas. Pancreas. 2012;41(2): 295–301.

Bae SY, Lee KT, Lee JH, et al. Proper management and follow-up strategy of branch duct intraductal papillary mucinous neoplasms of the pancreas. Dig Liver Dis. 2012;44(3):257–60.

Guarise A, Faccioli N, Ferrari M, et al. Evaluation of serial changes of pancreatic branch duct intraductal papillary mucinous neoplasms by follow-up with magnetic resonance imaging. Cancer Imaging. 2008;8:220–8.

Ikeuchi N, Itoi T, Sofuni A, et al. Prognosis of cancer with branch duct type IPMN of the pancreas. World J Gastroenterol. 2010;16(15):1890–5.

Ingakul T, Sadakari Y, Ienaga J, et al. Predictors of the presence of concomitant invasive ductal carcinoma in intraductal papillary mucinous neoplasm of the pancreas. Ann Surg. 2010;251(1):70–5.

Kang MJ, Jang JY, Kim SJ, et al. Cyst growth rate predicts malignancy in patients with branch duct intraductal papillary mucinous neoplasms. Clin Gastroentrol Hepatol. 2011;9(1):87–93.

Kanno A, Satoh K, Hirota M, et al. Prediction of invasive carcinoma in branch type intraductal papillary mucinous neoplasms of the pancreas. J Gastroenterol. 2010;45(9):952–9.

Khannoussi W, Vullierme MP, Rebours V, et al. The long term risk of malignancy in patients with branch duct intraductal papillary mucinous neoplasms of the pancreas. Pancreatology. 2012;12(3):198–202.

Kobayashi G, Fujita N, Noda Y, et al. Mode of progression of intraductal papillary-mucinous tumor of the pancreas: analysis of patients with follow-up by EUS. J Gastroenterol. 2005;40(7): 744–51.

Lee SH, Park JK, Woo SM, et al. Natural history of branch-duct type intraductal papillary mucinous neoplasms of the pancreas. Korean J Gastroenterol. 2007;49(1):24–30.

Maguchi H, Tanno S, Mizuno N, et al. Natural history of branch duct intraductal papillary mucinous neoplasms of the pancreas. A multicenter study in Japan. Pancreas. 2011;40(3):364–70.

Ohno E, Itoh A, Kawashima H, et al. Malignant transformation of branch duct-type intraductal papillary mucinous neoplasms of the pancreas based on contrast-enhanced endoscopic ultrasonography morphological changes: focus on malignant transformation of intraductal papillary mucinous neoplasm itself. Pancreas. 2012;41(6):855–62.

Pelaez-Luna M, Chari ST, Smyrk TC, et al. Do consensus indications for resection in branch duct intraductal papillary mucinous neoplasm predict malignancy? A study of 147 patients. Am J Gastroenterol. 2007;102(8):1759–64.

Rautou PE, Lévy P, Vullierme MP, et al. Morphologic changes in branch duct intraductal papillary mucinous neoplasms of the pancreas: a midterm follow-up study. Clin Gastroenterol Hepatol. 2008;6(7):807–14.

Rodriguez JR, Salvia R, Crippa S, et al. Branch-duct intraductal papillary mucinous neoplasms: observation in 145 patients who underwent resection. Gastroenterology. 2007;133(1):72–9.

Sawai Y, Yamao K, Bhatia V, et al. Development of pancreatic cancers during long-term follow-up of side-branch intraductal papillary mucinous neoplasms. Endoscopy. 2010;42(12):1077–84.

Tada M, Kawabe T, Arizumi M, et al. Pancreatic cancer in patients with pancreatic cystic lesions: a prospective study in 197 patients. Clin Gastroenterol Hepatol. 2006;4(10):1265–70.

Tanaka M, Chari S, Adsay V, et al. International consensus guidelines for management of intraductal papillary mucinous neoplasms and mucinous cystic neoplasms of the pancreas. Pancreatology. 2006;6(1–2):17–32.

Tanaka M, Castillo CF, Adsay V, et al. International consensus guideline 2012 for the management of IPMN and MCN of the pancreas. Pancreatology. 2012;12(3):183–97.

Tang RS, Weinberg B, Dawson DW, et al. Evaluation of the guidelines for management of pancreatic branch-duct intraductal papillary mucinous neoplasm. Clin Gastroenterol Hepatol. 2008;6(7):815–9.

Tanno S, Nakano Y, Nishikawa T, et al. Natural history of branch duct intraductal papillary-mucinous neoplasms of the pancreas without mural nodules: long-term follow-up results. Gut. 2008;57(3):339–43.

Tanno S, Nakano Y, Sugiyama Y, et al. Incidence of synchronous and metachronous pancreatic carcinoma in 168 patients with branch duct intraductal papillary mucinous neoplasm. Pancreatology. 2010a;10(2–3):173–8.

Tanno S, Nakano Y, Koizumi K, et al. Pancreatic ductal adenocarcinomas in long-term follow-up patients with branch duct intraductal papillary mucinous neoplasms. Pancreas. 2010b;39(1): 36–40.

Uehara H, Nakaizumi A, Ishikawa O, et al. Development of ductal carcinoma of the pancreas during follow-up of branch duct intraductal papillary mucinous neoplasm of the pancreas. Gut. 2008;57(11):1561–5.

Uehara H, Ishikawa O, Katayama K, et al. Size of mural nodule as an indicator of surgery for branch duct intraductal papillary mucinous neoplasm of the pancreas during follow-up. J Gastroenterol. 2011;46(5):657–63.

Yamaguchi K, Ohuchida J, Ohtsuka T, et al. Intraductal papillary-mucinous tumor of the pancreas concomitant with ductal carcinoma of the pancreas. Pancreatology. 2002;2(5):484–90.

Yamaguchi K, Kanemitsu S, Hatori T, et al. Pancreatic ductal adenocarcinoma derived from IPMN and pancreatic ductal adenocarcinoma concomitant with IPMN. Pancreas. 2011;40(4): 571–80.

Chapter 4
Histological Subclassification and Its Clinical Significance

Toru Furukawa

Abstract Intraductal papillary mucinous neoplasms (IPMNs) show variations in morphological and immunohistochemical features of cells and papillae. Based on the variations, IPMNs are classified into four distinct subtypes, namely, gastric type, intestinal type, pancreatobiliary type, and oncocytic type. These subtypes are well associated with clinicopathological features and known to be an independent prognostic factor. The gastric-type IPMNs show thick fingerlike papillae consisted of low-grade dysplastic cells expressing MUC5AC and occasionally MUC6. Patients with the gastric-type IPMN usually show fair prognosis. However, some of the gastric-type IPMNs are associated with invasive carcinoma that leads to poor prognosis. The intestinal-type IPMNs show villous papillae consisted of high-grade dysplastic cells expressing MUC2 and MUC5AC. They are often associated with mucinous colloid carcinoma. The prognosis is less favorable, around 90 % and 70 % in the 5- and 10-year survivals. The pancreatobiliary-type IPMNs show complex fernlike papillae consisted of high-grade dysplastic cells expressing MUC1 and MUC5AC. They are often associated with tubular adenocarcinoma and, hence, the prognosis is very poor, around 50 % and none in the 5- and 10-year survivals. The oncocytic-type IPMN show fractal-shaped papillae consisted of high-grade oncocytic cells expressing MUC5AC and MUC6. They are occasionally associated with oncocytic carcinoma. Prognosis is less favorable, around 80 % and 70 % in the 5- and 10-year survivals. These subtypes of IPMN can be determined not only on surgical specimen but also on cytology or biopsy specimen; hence, information of the subtypes is available during diagnostic process as well as postoperative follow-up, which is expected to facilitate better clinical management of patients with IPMN.

Keywords Gastric type • Intestinal type • Oncocytic type • Pancreatobiliary type

T. Furukawa (✉)
Institute for Integrated Medical Sciences, Tokyo Women's Medical University, Tokyo, Japan
e-mail: furukawa.toru@twmu.ac.jp

M. Tanaka (ed.), *Intraductal Papillary Mucinous Neoplasm of the Pancreas*,
DOI 10.1007/978-4-431-54472-2_4, © Springer Japan 2014

4.1 Introductory Remarks

The intraductal papillary mucinous neoplasm (IPMN) is characterized by dilated ducts filled with mucin (Adsay et al. 2010). Neoplastic cells line inner surface of the dilated duct and show papillae with diverse morphologic features and various degree of atypia. IPMN was firstly reported as a distinctive pancreatic neoplasm in 1982 by Ohhashi et al. (1982). Since this first report, a number of reports have been published, initially from Japan mostly and later from Western countries as well, and the term IPMN has been coined and described in World Health Organization Classification of Tumours (Klöppel et al. 1996). As many cases are being accumulated, it has become obvious that IPMNs include a spectrum of neoplasms with both morphological and immunohistochemical variations of cells and papillae. The morphological variations regard histological features of cells including nuclear size and shape and cytoplasmic appearance and shapes of papillae showing fingerlike, villous, ferny, or fractal. The immunohistochemical variations regard mucin proteins aberrantly expressed in neoplastic cells including MUC1, MUC2, MUC5AC, and MUC6. Yonezawa et al. described in their pioneering study of 24 cases of IPMN that histological variations of IPMNs could be classified into three distinct types, namely, villous dark cell type, papillary clear cell type, and compact cell type (Yonezawa et al. 1999). Adsay et al. introduced 11 cases of intraductal oncocytic papillary neoplasms (Adsay et al. 1996) and also classified variants of other 74 IPMNs into three types including intestinal type, pancreatobiliary type, and null type (Adsay et al. 2002, 2004). Based on these studies and a consensus meeting held on 2003, Furukawa et al. published the consensus classification of the variations of IPMN into four distinct subtypes, namely, gastric type, intestinal type, pancreatobiliary type, and oncocytic type (Furukawa et al. 2005b). These subtypes have become evident to be associated with distinct clinicopathological features including prognosis in patients with IPMN (Furukawa et al. 2011a; Kim et al. 2011).

4.2 Pathology of IPMN

IPMN is a neoplasm arising in the inner surface of pancreatic duct (Furukawa et al. 1992). It consists of tall columnar cells secreting mucin. The cells show various degree of atypia manifested by nuclear enlargement, irregular nuclear shape, hyperchromatism, coarse chromatin, nucleoli prominence, increasing of nucleocytoplasmic ratio, nuclear stratification, and loss of polarity. Mucin is abundant in cytoplasm and is composed of various glycoproteins including MUC1, MUC2, MUC5AC, and MUC6. MUC1 is a component of the membrane-bound type of mucin and is detected in luminal surfaces of acini in the normal pancreas (Abe and Kufe 1993). MUC2 consists of secreted mucin usually observed in intestinal glands. MUC2 is considered to be a marker of intestinal differentiation and not expressed in the normal pancreas (Gum et al. 1989). MUC5AC is expressed in mucous surface cells of the stomach. MUC5AC is not detected in the normal pancreas but is consistently detected in IPMNs and pancreatic intraepithelial neoplasia (PanIN), a precursor lesion associated with invasive ductal adenocarcinoma (Yonezawa et al. 1999; Kim et al. 2002). MUC6 is secretary mucin expressed commonly in gastric pyloric glands and duodenal Brunner's glands and occasionally in small intralobular ducts in the pancreas (Bartman et al. 1998). The cells of IPMN comprise papillae in various shapes and size, which are thick fingerlike, villous, fernlike, or fractal. Some portions of a neoplasm can be flat with tall columnar cells. Differences in the shapes of papillae and immunohistochemical features of expressed MUC proteins in neoplastic cells are principal features for subclassification of IPMN as described below. IPMN is graded by degree of atypia into low grade, moderate grade, or high grade (Adsay et al. 2010). Low- or moderate-grade neoplasms are regarded as adenoma while high-grade neoplasms are regarded as carcinoma (noninvasive). Approximately 30 % of IPMNs have invasion, and such cases are designated as IPMN with an associated invasive carcinoma (Adsay et al. 2010). The invasive carcinoma associated with IPMN is histologically either tubular, colloid, or oncocytic. Tubular adenocarcinoma associated with IPMN is similar to conventional ductal adenocarcinoma of the pancreas showing invasive tubular glands in desmoplastic stroma. Conversely, ductal adenocarcinoma with cystic ducts with papillary proliferation of epithelial cells shown inside should be carefully evaluated whether it is associated with IPMN or not. Colloid carcinoma associated with IPMN shows mucus lakes with floating clusters of neoplastic cells in adjacent stroma of dilated ducts. Oncocytic carcinoma associated with IPMN shows invasive oncocytic cell clusters in stroma. Occasionally, penetration of dilated ducts with abundant mucinous content into adjacent duodenum or bile duct can be seen, even without obvious cellular invasion. IPMNs involving the main duct are called the main duct type, those involving branch ducts are called the branch duct type, and those involving both ducts are called the mixed type. These features of differential involvement of ducts can be assessed in clinical imaging studies and noted as important features for managing patients with IPMN as described elsewhere in this book. Theoretically, IPMNs with high-grade dysplasia and those with an associated invasive carcinoma should be completely resected. For the complete resection, frozen section diagnosis is employed for assessing surgical margin. Surgical margin involved with invasive carcinoma or high-grade dysplasia should be further resected if the additional resection will be tolerated by the patient. Surgical margin with low- or moderate-grade dysplasia can be dismissed without further resection (Tanaka et al. 2012). Staging is made according to TNM staging system described in the American Joint Committee on Cancer (AJCC) Staging Handbook (Greene et al. 2002). Furukawa et al. proposed an additional special modification of AJCC for staging IPMNs with defining IPMNs with low- or moderate-grade dysplasia as Tisa and TisaN0M0 as stage 0A (Furukawa et al. 2011a).

4.3 Histological Subclassification of IPMN

The classification of histological variations of IPMN into four subtypes including the gastric type, the intestinal type, the pancreatobiliary type, and the oncocytic type is based on histomorphological and immunohistochemical features as summarized (Table 4.1 and Fig. 4.1).

Table 4.1 Subtypes of intraductal papillary mucinous neoplasm of the pancreas

Subtype	Mimicker	Criteria	Atypia	MUC1	MUC2	MUC5AC	MUC6
Gastric	Foveolae	Low grade: thick fingerlike papillae consisted of cells with amphophilic cytoplasm and basally located small nuclei High grade: irregular low-height papillae consisted of cells with enlarged nuclei with coarse chromatin and high nucleocytoplasmic ratio	Low or high grade	–	–	+	–
	Pyloric gland	Polypoid papillae consisted of tubular glands. Cells have amphophilic cytoplasm and small, round, and basally located nuclei	Low grade	–	–	+	+
Intestinal	Villous neoplasm	Villous papillae consisted of cells with basophilic cytoplasm and enlarged cigar-shaped nuclei with dense chromatin, pseudostratification, and loss of polarity	Moderate or high grade	–	+	+	–
Pancreatobiliary	Cholangiopapillary neoplasm	Arborizing complex fernlike papillae consisted of cells with enlarged and irregular-shaped nuclei with coarse chromatin, amphophilic cytoplasm, and high nucleocytoplasmic ratio	High grade	+	–	+	+ or –
Oncocytic	Oncocytic neoplasm	Thick branching fractal-shaped papillae with intracellular and intraepithelial lumina consisted of cells with eosinophilic cytoplasm, large round nuclei with prominent nucleoli, and high nucleocytoplasmic ratio	High grade	+ or –	+ or –	+	+

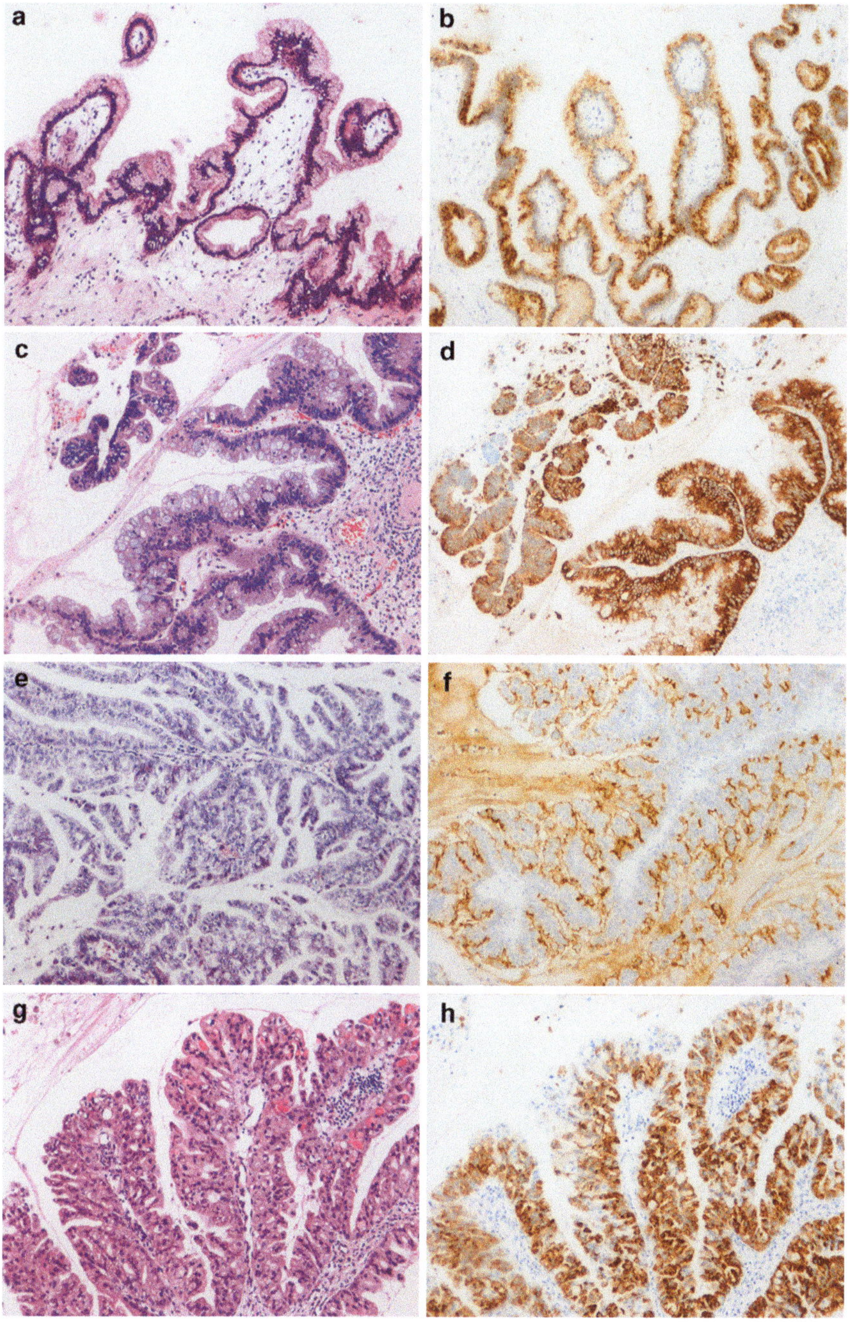

Fig. 4.1 Subtypes of IPMN. (**a**) and (**b**). Gastric-type IPMN consisted of thick fingerlike papillae resembling gastric foveolae (**a**) labeled with anti-MUC5AC (**b**). (**c**) and (**d**). Intestinal-type IPMN consisted of villous papillae resembling intestinal villous neoplasms (**c**) labeled with anti-MUC2 (**d**). (**e**) and (**f**). Pancreatobiliary-type IPMN consisted of arborizing complex fernlike papillae resembling cholangiopapillary carcinoma (**e**) labeled with anti-MUC1 (**f**). (**g**) and (**h**). Oncocytic-type IPMN consisted of thick fractal-shaped papillae with eosinophilic cells (**g**) labeled with anti-MUC6 (**h**). (**a**), (**c**), (**e**), and (**g**): Hematoxylin and eosin staining. (**b**), (**d**), (**f**), and (**h**): Immunohistochemistry with diaminobenzidine as a chromogen. Original magnification of all panels is ×100

4.3.1 Gastric-Type IPMN

The gastric-type IPMN shows thick fingerlike papillae resembling gastric foveolae (Fig. 4.1a). Nuclei of neoplastic cells are usually round and small and show fine chromatin and preserved polarity, which corresponds to low-grade dysplasia that leads to a diagnosis of adenoma. Cytoplasm is abundant and amphophilic and labeled with anti-MUC5AC antibody by immunohistochemistry but not with anti-MUC1 or anti-MUC2 (Fig. 4.1b). The null type or the clear cell type of IPMN previously reported corresponds to the gastric-type IPMN (Adsay et al. 2004; Yonezawa et al. 1999). Occasionally, the neoplasm is consisted of glands resembling pyloric glands that form a polypoid lesion in the dilated duct (Fig. 4.2a). Cells of this pyloric-gland subtype are labeled with anti-MUC5AC and anti-MUC6 but not with anti-MUC1 or anti-MUC2. Notably, around 20 % of gastric-type IPMNs can present with highly atypical cells with irregular large nuclei with coarse chromatin and loss of polarity consisting papillae in irregular shape and low height (Furukawa et al. 2011a) (Fig. 4.2b). This high-grade gastric-type IPMNs are often associated with invasive tubular adenocarcinoma and show poor prognosis as described later.

4.3.2 Intestinal-Type IPMN

The intestinal-type IPMN shows villous papillae consisted of pseudostratified tall columnar cells with large and oval, often cigar-shaped, nuclei with dense chromatin and obvious nucleoli, which resembles an intestinal villous neoplasm (Fig. 4.1c). Cytoplasm is somewhat basophilic and contains abundant mucin droplets. These cellular features correspond to high-grade dysplasia, which leads to a diagnosis of intraductal carcinoma. Some areas of the neoplasm are composed of cells showing goblet cell appearance with low-grade atypia (Fig. 4.2c). Neoplastic cells of the intestinal type secrete thick copious mucin and are labeled with anti-MUC2 and anti-MUC5AC but not with anti-MUC1 or anti-MUC6 (Fig. 4.1d). The dark cell type of IPMN previously reported corresponds to the intestinal-type IPMN (Yonezawa et al. 1999). The intestinal-type IPMN is often associated with colloid mucinous carcinoma showing mucinous lakes with floating epithelial clusters in stroma (Fig. 4.2d). Rarely, mucinous content penetrates from the pancreatic duct into adjacent duodenum or bile duct even without obvious cellular invasion.

4.3.3 Pancreatobiliary-Type IPMN

The pancreatobiliary-type IPMN shows tall, complex, and arborizing fernlike papillae resembling cholangiopapillary neoplasm (Fig. 4.1e). Cells consisting of the papillae show large irregular nuclei with coarse chromatin and prominent nucleoli

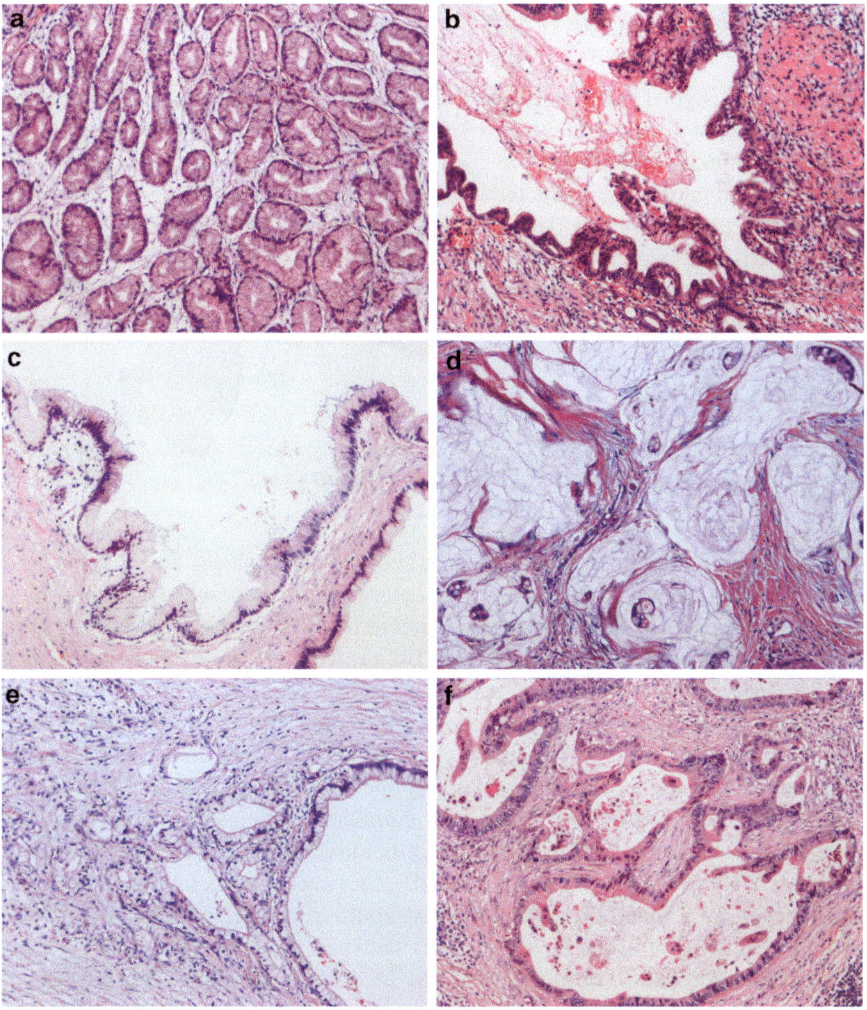

Fig. 4.2 Variation of IPMN subtypes. (**a**) Gastric-type IPMN with pyloric-like glands. (**b**) Gastric-type IPMN with high-grade dysplasia. (**c**) Intestinal-type IPMN with goblet cell like low-grade dysplasia. (**d**) Colloid carcinoma associated with IPMN. (**e**) Tubular adenocarcinoma associated with IPMN. (**f**) Oncocytic carcinoma associated with IPMN. All panels are hematoxylin and eosin staining. Original magnification is ×100

in scarce cytoplasm, loss of polarity, and high nucleocytoplasmic ratio, which leads to a diagnosis of high-grade dysplasia or intraductal carcinoma. Moreover, this type is often associated with invasive tubular adenocarcinoma that is similar to the conventional type of pancreatic cancer (Fig. 4.2e). The pancreatobiliary-type IPMN is labeled with anti-MUC1 and anti-MUC5AC, occasionally with anti-MUC6, but not with anti-MUC2 (Fig. 4.1f).

4.3.4 Oncocytic-Type IPMN

The oncocytic-type IPMN is consisted of oncocytic cells forming thick branching papillae often in fractal shape (Fig. 4.1g). The cells contain large round nuclei with coarse chromatin in eosinophilic cytoplasm. Loss of polarity is obvious and intraepithelial lumina are characteristic. These features indicate high-grade dysplasia or intraductal carcinoma. The cells are labeled consistently with anti-MUC5AC and anti-MUC6, and occasionally with anti-MUC1 or anti-MUC2 (Fig. 4.1h). Sometimes oncocytic cells are seen invasive in surrounding stroma of dilated duct, and the invasive component is assessed as an associated oncocytic carcinoma (Fig. 4.2f).

4.3.5 Interpretation of the Subtypes of IPMN

In pathological examination, IPMNs are subtyped based on the above-mentioned morphological criteria, which usually is not a difficult task because the morphological features are obvious and characteristic (Furukawa et al. 2005b). Immunohistochemical examination of MUC proteins greatly helps to assess and confirm the subtyping, which is especially useful for atypical cases. The subtyping is possible on biopsy or even in cytology specimen (Hibi et al. 2007; Hara et al. 2013). IPMNs often are composed of a combination of more than one neoplastic subtype, usually the gastric type and either one of other types. When several subtypes are recognized in one IPMN, the dominant component should be documented as a represented subtype with any other less significant subtypes. In a case of invasive carcinoma associated with IPMN, the subtype of an intraductal component as well as a histological phenotype of invasive cancer should be noted with special attention on areas of associations between the intraductal and invasive components (Furukawa et al. 2005b). The invasive component should be documented with an appropriate grading and staging as done for conventional pancreatic ductal adenocarcinoma (PDA). The low-grade gastric-type component is often seen multiple and accompanies with other high-grade components. Conversely, the high-grade neoplasms, either intestinal, pancreatobiliary, or oncocytic, often form one united lesion with peripheral or surrounding multiple low-grade gastric lesions (Furukawa et al. 1992). This implies that the low-grade gastric neoplasm may be a precursor of other types of neoplasms; hence, high-grade IPMNs would be a result of progression of the low-grade gastric-type IPMN, which, although somewhat apparent, has not been experimentally proved yet. Nevertheless, this assumption could be crucial for management of IPMN because the low-grade gastric IPMN is supposed to undergo surveillance for progression, which is indeed recommended in the current consensus guideline for management of patients with IPMN (Tanaka et al. 2012).

4.4 Clinicopathological Features Characteristic for the Subtypes of IPMN

The subtypes are well associated with clinicopathological features of patients with IPMN (Furukawa et al. 2011a; Kim et al. 2011).

4.4.1 *Clinicopathological Features of Gastric-Type IPMN*

Gastric-type IPMNs usually show low-grade dysplasia and are assessed as adenoma. The neoplasm predominantly involves branching ducts, which leads to form relatively small cysts, often multiple, in the pancreas. Conversely, small cysts are likely to be gastric-type IPMNs with low-grade dysplasia, and these lesions can be observed with appropriate cautions (Tanaka et al. 2012). The prognosis is fair when resected, over 90 % in the 5- and 10-year survival rates. Hence most of the gastric-type IPMNs can be regarded as "benign" neoplasms; however, notably in a retrospective study with 182 surgically treated patients (Furukawa et al. 2011a), 5 % of patients with gastric-type IPMNs died of the disease; these patients had high-grade dysplastic neoplasms with an associated invasive tubular adenocarcinoma. This indicates that although most of patients with the gastric-type IPMN have benign phenotypes and fair prognoses, some patients develop high-grade neoplasms likely to be associated with invasive carcinoma that leads them to poor prognosis.

4.4.2 *Clinicopathological Features of Intestinal-Type IPMN*

Intestinal-type IPMNs usually have villous complex papillae showing high-grade dysplasia. The neoplasms often involve the main duct, which reveals marked dilatation of the duct with abundant mucin. Occasionally, the neoplasm involves the main duct mostly or entirely, which necessitates total pancreatectomy for complete resection (Tanaka et al. 2012; Furukawa et al. 1992). Around 50 % of the neoplasms are invasive and the invasion shows almost always mucinous colloid feature (Adsay et al. 2004; Furukawa et al. 2011a; Kim et al. 2011). Conversely, mucinous colloid carcinoma is exclusively associated with the intestinal-type IPMN. The prognosis of patients with intestinal IPMN is less favorable, around 90 % and 70 % in the 5- and 10-year survival rates, respectively (Adsay et al. 2004; Furukawa et al. 2011a; Kim et al. 2011). Intestinal IPMNs with an associated invasive carcinoma show 70 % and 50 % in 5- and 10-year survivals, respectively (Furukawa et al. 2011a). Some patients with noninvasive high-grade intestinal-type IPMNs develop a recurrent tumor even after initial complete resection in long-term follow-up, which is uncommon in other types of IPMN (Furukawa et al. 2011a). The recurrence could originally be a residual multifocal or skip tumor unrecognized at the time of initial surgery or correspond to a metachronous development of IPMN. This indicates importance of postoperative surveillance to find recurrence.

4.4.3 Clinicopathological Features of Pancreatobiliary-Type IPMN

Pancreatobiliary-type IPMNs exclusively show high-grade atypia and are often, 57–77 %, associated with invasive tubular adenocarcinoma (Adsay et al. 2004; Furukawa et al. 2011a; Kim et al. 2011). They do not show any preference for involving portion of duct. Patient prognosis is around 50 % and 0 % in the 5- and 10-year survival rates, respectively, which is the poorest among the subtypes of IPMN (Adsay et al. 2004; Furukawa et al. 2011a; Kim et al. 2011). This very poor prognosis can account for the high susceptibility of this IPMN type to develop invasive tubular adenocarcinoma. Indeed, in our previous study including 12 cases with invasive pancreatobiliary-type IPMNs, no patients of 5-year survival were obtained (Furukawa et al. 2011a). However, noninvasive pancreatobiliary-type IPMNs can have a fair prognosis, which emphasizes the importance of early diagnosis of the pancreatobiliary-type IPMN (Furukawa et al. 2011a).

4.4.4 Clinicopathological Features of Oncocytic-Type IPMN

Oncocytic-type IPMNs are least common among the four types of IPMN and tend to occur in a relatively younger people than other types of IPMN (Furukawa et al. 2011a; Kim et al. 2011). The neoplasm usually involves branch duct, which forms a well-developed cyst with solid component. However notably, it often extends into surrounding connecting ductal surface with little dilatation. The neoplasms show high-grade dysplasia, and around 50 % of them are associated with invasive carcinoma showing oncocytic feature, often limited in small area (Adsay et al. 2004; Furukawa et al. 2011a; Kim et al. 2011). The patients with oncocytic-type IPMNs have less favorable prognosis, around 80 % and 70 % in the 5- and 10-year survival rates, respectively (Adsay et al. 2004; Furukawa et al. 2011a; Kim et al. 2011). Those with invasive oncocytic IPMNs reveal 60 % and 40 % in 5- and 10-year survivals, respectively (Furukawa et al. 2011a).

4.5 Molecular Pathology and the Subtypes of IPMN

4.5.1 GNAS

Recent studies have uncovered that *GNAS* is frequently and specifically mutated in IPMNs. *GNAS* is found mutated in 46–65 % of IPMNs and the mutations exclusively occur at codon 201, mostly are R201H or R201C (Furukawa et al. 2011b; Wu et al. 2011b). Strikingly, *GNAS* mutations have never been found in PDA, a conventional type of pancreatic cancer. This indicates that *GNAS* mutation is quite common and highly specific for IPMN (Furukawa et al. 2011b; Wu et al. 2011b). *GNAS* encodes

G-protein alpha subunit (Gsα) that is a mediator in G-protein coupled receptor (GPCR) signaling pathway (Landis et al. 1989). Gsα forms a heterotrimer with β and γ G-protein subunits, which then couple with a membrane-bound receptor, GPCR. When GPCR is activated by ligand binding, the receptor catalyzes exchange of guanosine triphosphate (GTP) for guanosine diphosphate (GDP) bound to Gsα, and the GTP-bound Gsα dissociates from the receptor and the βγ subunits. The dissociated Gsα proceeds to activate specific effector molecules including adenyl cyclase, which produces cyclic AMP (cAMP) that can act as a second messenger (Dhanasekaran 2006). Increased cAMP activates cAMP-dependent protein kinase (PKA), and the activated PKA phosphorylates variety of target molecules. Gsα has an intrinsic hydrolase activity that converts GTP to GDP and the active GTP-bound Gsa turns into the inactive GDP-bound form. R201H and R201C mutations in *GNAS* result in abolishing this intrinsic hydrolase activity, which leads to constitutive activation of Gsα and its downstream cascades (Landis et al. 1989). *GNAS* mutations are found in no matter what grade of IPMN, i.e., from low grade to high grade and invasive, which may indicate that *GNAS* mutation or activation of Gsα is necessary for development of IPMN (Furukawa et al. 2011b). Moreover, although the mutation is found in all of the four subtypes of IPMN, it is more common in intestinal-type IPMNs than any other types. This suggests that *GNAS* mutation may contribute to and be selected in development or progression into the intestinal-type IPMNs. Functional roles of *GNAS* mutation or activation of Gsα in development and progression of IPMN remain to be explored.

4.5.2 RNF43

RNF43 is also just recently discovered to be mutated in IPMNs by whole exome sequencing (Furukawa et al. 2011b; Wu et al. 2011a). Most of mutations in *RNF43* so far found in IPMNs have been either nonsense or frameshift mutations. The nonsense or frameshift mutation usually results in generation of a truncated, often nonfunctioning, protein, which corresponds to a loss-of-function mutation commonly found in tumor suppressor genes. Hence, *RNF43* is supposed to be a tumor suppressor gene, i.e., a gatekeeper for IPMN. Interestingly, *RNF43* mutation has been found not in PDA but in mucinous cystic neoplasms (MCN) of the pancreas, which indicates that *RNF43* is a susceptible gene for mucinous neoplasms including IPMN and MCN but not for the conventional solid type of pancreatic cancer (Wu et al. 2011a). *RNF43* encodes ring finger protein 43, an ubiquitin ligase. Ubiquitin ligase functions to bind ubiquitin to target proteins for letting them to proteosomal degradation. The target protein so far identified for ring finger protein 43 is FZD5, the frizzled receptor important for provoking WNT signaling transduction, which indicates that ring finger protein 43 functions to control WNT signaling activity (Koo et al. 2012). The loss-of-function mutation in *RNF43* would result in aberrant activation of WNT signaling and may contribute to development and progression of IPMN. Associations between *RNF43* mutation and clinicopathological phenotypes of IPMN including morphological types are issues to be studied.

4.5.3 *KRAS*

Mutations in *KRAS* are found in 50–80 % of IPMNs (Hoshi et al. 1994; Satoh et al. 1996), less common than those in PDA, in which the mutations are found in 80–90 % of them (Almoguera et al. 1988; Caldas and Kern 1995). *KRAS* encodes rat sarcoma oncogene homologue protein (RAS) and the RAS is a signal transmitter in the receptor tyrosine kinase (RTK) signaling pathway (Thatcher 2010). One of the RTK pathways that primarily function in the pancreatic neoplasms is the mitogen-activated protein kinase (MAPK) pathway. RAS is activated by binding with GTP and it has an intrinsic hydrolase activity to convert GTP to GDP and to turn itself inactive, just as Gsα. Mutation in *KRAS* occur at codon 12, 13, and 61, which can abolish the hydrolase activity of RAS and make RAS constitutively active, again just like mutant *GNAS*. Mutations in *KRAS* are associated not with grade but with the subtype of IPMN. Gastric- and pancreatobiliary-type IPMNs are more likely to harbor *KRAS* mutation than intestinal- and oncocytic-type IPMNs (Furukawa et al. 2011b). Oncocytic-type IPMNs harbor *KRAS* mutations in exceptionally low frequency among the types, 17 % of them, which indicates that the oncocytic IPMNs may develop by distinct molecular mechanisms yet undetermined (Xiao et al. 2011). Mutations in *KRAS* are more frequently observed than *GNAS* in IPMNs. Moreover, mutation in *GNAS* and *KRAS* can be found simultaneously in IPMNs, 25–50 % of them. The overlapping mutations do not seem to be associated with any specific clinicopathological features (Furukawa et al. 2011b; Wu et al. 2011b). Whether mutations in *KRAS* and *GNAS* would function independently or synergistically is an important issue to be answered.

4.5.4 Other Molecules Associated with IPMN

Mutations in *PIK3CA* are found in a few IPMNs (Schönleben et al. 2006). *PIK3CA* mutations usually occur at codon 545 or 1047. *PIK3CA* encodes p110-alpha, a 110 kDa catalytic subunit, comprising phosphatidylinositol 3-kinase. p110-alpha is composed of a helical domain and a kinase domain, in which E545K affects the helical domain and H1047R and G1049R affect the kinase domain (Samuels et al. 2004). Studies have proved that p110-alpha of E545K and that of H1047R are both functionally active (Samuels et al. 2004). Although *PIK3CA* mutations are rare in IPMN, they may be common in the intraductal tubulopapillary neoplasm of the pancreas, another type of intraductal pancreatic neoplasm (Yamaguchi et al. 2011).

Expression of cyclin-dependent kinase inhibitor 2a (CDKN2A) is lost in 10–50 % of low-grade IPMNs and 80–100 % of high-grade IPMNs (Furukawa et al. 2005a; Biankin et al. 2002). The loss of expression is due to genetic deletion or epigenetic alterations, in which the latter, mostly hypermethylation of a promoter region of its encoding gene, *CDKN2A*, seems to be common in IPMN (House et al. 2003). CDKN2A plays a role in arresting the cell cycle progression. Loss of function of

CDKN2A leads to abnormal cell cycle progression and cell proliferation (Serrano et al. 1993). The loss of expression is not specifically associated with the subtypes of IPMN (Mohri et al. 2012).

Tumor protein 53 (TP53) is aberrantly expressed in 20 % of high-grade IPMNs and invasive carcinoma associated with IPMN (Furukawa et al. 2005a; Sasaki et al. 2003). The aberrant expression can be observed as nuclear accumulation or loss of expression. TP53 is a transcription factor responding to DNA damage and functions to protect genome integrity. Loss of function of TP53 leads to genome instability and contributes to tumorigenesis (Gerwin et al. 1992). The aberrant expression of TP53 is significantly more often observed in pancreatobiliary-type IPMNs (Kuboki and Furukawa, unpublished data).

Expression of Sma- and Mad-related protein 4 (SMAD4) is retained in noninvasive IPMNs but lost in some of invasive carcinomas associated with IPMN (Biankin et al. 2002). SMAD4 is a mediator in the signaling cascade evoked by transforming growth factor beta, which is associated with a variety of functions including differentiation, cell motility, phenotypic transition, proliferation, and stem cell features (Morikawa et al. 2012). Loss of expression of SMAD4 is common in PDAs, 50–90 % of them, and the loss is caused by genetic deletion or mutation (Hahn et al. 1996; Furukawa et al. 2005a). The loss of expression of SMAD4 seems to be more common in pancreatobiliary-type than other type of IPMNs (Kuboki and Furukawa, unpublished data).

4.6 The Subtype of IPMN and Clinical Management

The current recommendations for the diagnostic and preoperative management of IPMN patients depend on assessment of clinical features designated as "high-risk stigmata" and "worrisome features." "High-risk stigmata" include the following features: (1) obstructive jaundice in a patient with cystic lesion of the head of the pancreas, (2) enhancing solid component within cyst, and (3) main pancreatic duct >10 mm in size. "Worrisome features" include (1) cyst >3 cm, (2) thickened/enhancing cyst walls, (3) main duct size 5–9 mm, (4) non-enhancing mural nodule, and (5) abrupt change in caliber of pancreatic duct with distal pancreatic atrophy (Tanaka et al. 2012). Patients with "high-risk stigmata" are recommended to undergo surgery and those with "worrisome features" may be followed with appropriate medical surveillance examinations. Hence, the size of the lesion, the differential involvement of ducts (main or branch), and the presence of mural nodules are regarded as key features to determine clinical management of patients with IPMN. In addition to these features, information of the subtypes of IPMN may help to design more appropriate management because the subtype is not only well associated with these key features but also an independent strong prognostic value (Furukawa et al. 2011a). During the diagnostic process, subtype of IPMN can be determined on cytology or biopsy specimen (Hibi et al. 2007; Hara et al. 2013). By obtaining information of subtypes of IPMN, clinical management could be more appropriately determined. For example, a gastric-type IPMN has usually localized but often multiple low-grade lesions; an intestinal-type IPMN tends to form a diffuse high-grade lesion involving the main duct, often invasive, and has considerable probability of recurrence; a pancreatobiliary-type IPMN is likely to have an invasive lesion of tubular adenocarcinoma; and an oncocytic-type IPMN may extend into ducts without dilatation and have a small invasive lesion. Thus comparing the information of the subtypes and clinical imaging, surgery can be designed as a limited pancreatectomy for removal of a localized gastric-type IPMN; an extensive, and often total, pancreatectomy for an intestinal-type IPMN; a radical pancreatectomy for a pancreatobiliary-type IPMN; and a standard pancreatectomy for an oncocytic-type IPMN. The high risk of disease-specific death due to invasive pancreatobiliary-type IPMNs may illustrate the requirement for adjuvant therapy as a conventional PDA. For follow-up surveillance, not only invasive IPMNs but also noninvasive intestinal-type IPMN should be carefully examined for recurrence (Furukawa et al. 2011a). Therefore, information of the subtypes is available during diagnostic process and follow-up, which is expected to facilitate better clinical management of patients with IPMN.

References

Abe M, Kufe D. Characterization of cis-acting elements regulating transcription of the human DF3 breast carcinoma-associated antigen (MUC1) gene. Proc Natl Acad Sci U S A. 1993;90(1): 282–6.

Adsay NV, Adair CF, Heffess CS, Klimstra DS. Intraductal oncocytic papillary neoplasms of the pancreas. Am J Surg Pathol. 1996;20(8):980–94.

Adsay NV, Conlon KC, Zee SY, Brennan MF, Klimstra DS. Intraductal papillary-mucinous neoplasms of the pancreas: an analysis of in situ and invasive carcinomas in 28 patients. Cancer. 2002;94(1):62–77.

Adsay NV, Merati K, Basturk O, Iacobuzio-Donahue C, Levi E, Cheng JD, et al. Pathologically and biologically distinct types of epithelium in intraductal papillary mucinous neoplasms: delineation of an "intestinal" pathway of carcinogenesis in the pancreas. Am J Surg Pathol. 2004;28(7):839–48.

Adsay NV, Fukushima N, Furukawa T, Hruban RH, Klimstra DS, Klöppel G, et al. Intraductal neoplasms of the pancreas. In: Bosman FT, Hruban RH, Carneiro F, Theise ND, editors. WHO classification of tumours of the digestive system. WHO classification of tumours. 4th ed. Lyon: IARC; 2010. p. 304–13.

Almoguera C, Shibata D, Forrester K, Martin J, Arnheim N, Perucho M. Most human carcinomas of the exocrine pancreas contain mutant c-K-ras genes. Cell. 1988;53(4):549–54.

Bartman AE, Buisine MP, Aubert JP, Niehans GA, Toribara NW, Kim YS, et al. The MUC6 secretory mucin gene is expressed in a wide variety of epithelial tissues. J Pathol. 1998;186(4):398–405.

Biankin AV, Biankin SA, Kench JG, Morey AL, Lee CS, Head DR, et al. Aberrant p16(INK4A) and DPC4/Smad4 expression in intraductal papillary mucinous tumours of the pancreas is associated with invasive ductal adenocarcinoma. Gut. 2002;50(6):861–8.

Caldas C, Kern SE. K-ras mutation and pancreatic adenocarcinoma. Int J Pancreatol. 1995; 18(1):1–6.

Dhanasekaran DN. Transducing the signals: a G protein takes a new identity. Sci STKE. 2006; 2006(347):pe31.

Furukawa T, Takahashi T, Kobari M, Matsuno S. The mucus-hypersecreting tumor of the pancreas. Development and extension visualized by three-dimensional computerized mapping. Cancer. 1992;70(6):1505–13.

Furukawa T, Fujisaki R, Yoshida Y, Kanai N, Sunamura M, Abe T, et al. Distinct progression pathways involving the dysfunction of DUSP6/MKP-3 in pancreatic intraepithelial neoplasia and intraductal papillary-mucinous neoplasms of the pancreas. Mod Pathol. 2005a;18(8):1034–42.

Furukawa T, Kloppel G, Volkan Adsay N, Albores-Saavedra J, Fukushima N, Horii A, et al. Classification of types of intraductal papillary-mucinous neoplasm of the pancreas: a consensus study. Virchows Arch. 2005b;447(5):794–9.

Furukawa T, Hatori T, Fujita I, Yamamoto M, Kobayashi M, Ohike N, et al. Prognostic relevance of morphological types of intraductal papillary mucinous neoplasms of the pancreas. Gut. 2011a;60(4):509–16.

Furukawa T, Kuboki Y, Tanji E, Yoshida S, Hatori T, Yamamoto M, et al. Whole-exome sequencing uncovers frequent GNAS mutations in intraductal papillary mucinous neoplasms of the pancreas. Sci Rep. 2011b;1:161.

Gerwin BI, Spillare E, Forrester K, Lehman TA, Kispert J, Welsh JA, et al. Mutant p53 can induce tumorigenic conversion of human bronchial epithelial cells and reduce their responsiveness to a negative growth factor, transforming growth factor beta 1. Proc Natl Acad Sci U S A. 1992;89(7):2759–63.

Greene FL, Page DL, Fleming ID, Fritz A, Balch CM. AJCC cancer staging handbook. 6th ed. New York: Springer; 2002.

Gum JR, Byrd JC, Hicks JW, Toribara NW, Lamport DT, Kim YS. Molecular cloning of human intestinal mucin cDNAs. Sequence analysis and evidence for genetic polymorphism. J Biol Chem. 1989;264(11):6480–7.

Hahn SA, Schutte M, Hoque AT, Moskaluk CA, da Costa LT, Rozenblum E, et al. DPC4, a candidate tumor suppressor gene at human chromosome 18q21.1. Science. 1996;271(5247):350–3.

Hara T, Ikebe D, Odaka A, Sudo K, Nakamura K, Yamamoto H, Itami M, Hirata T, Kashimura J, Yamaguchi T. Preoperative histological subtype classification of intraductal papillary mucinous neoplasms (IPMN) by pancreatic juice cytology with MUC stain. Ann Surg. 2013. doi: 10.1097/SLA.0b013e318281b824.

Hibi Y, Fukushima N, Tsuchida A, Sofuni A, Itoi T, Moriyasu F, et al. Pancreatic juice cytology and subclassification of intraductal papillary mucinous neoplasms of the pancreas. Pancreas. 2007;34(2):197–204.

Hoshi T, Imai M, Ogawa K. Frequent K-ras mutations and absence of p53 mutations in mucin-producing tumors of the pancreas. J Surg Oncol. 1994;55(2):84–91.

House MG, Guo M, Iacobuzio-Donahue C, Herman JG. Molecular progression of promoter methylation in intraductal papillary mucinous neoplasms (IPMN) of the pancreas. Carcinogenesis. 2003;24(2):193–8.

Kim GE, Bae HI, Park HU, Kuan SF, Crawley SC, Ho JJ, et al. Aberrant expression of MUC5AC and MUC6 gastric mucins and sialyl Tn antigen in intraepithelial neoplasms of the pancreas. Gastroenterol. 2002;123(4):1052–60.

Kim J, Jang KT, Mo Park S, Lim SW, Kim JH, Lee KH, et al. Prognostic relevance of pathologic subtypes and minimal invasion in intraductal papillary mucinous neoplasms of the pancreas. Tumour Biol. 2011;32(3):535–42. doi:10.1007/s13277-010-0148-z.

Klöppel G, Solcia E, Longnecker DS, Capella C, Sobin LH. Histological typing of tumours of the exocrine pancreas. International histological classification of tumours. 2nd ed. Berlin: Springer; 1996.

Koo BK, Spit M, Jordens I, Low TY, Stange DE, van de Wetering M, et al. Tumour suppressor RNF43 is a stem-cell E3 ligase that induces endocytosis of Wnt receptors. Nature. 2012; 488(7413):665–9.

Landis CA, Masters SB, Spada A, Pace AM, Bourne HR, Vallar L. GTPase inhibiting mutations activate the alpha chain of Gs and stimulate adenylyl cyclase in human pituitary tumours. Nature. 1989;340(6236):692–6.

Mohri D, Asaoka Y, Ijichi H, Miyabayashi K, Kudo Y, Seto M, et al. Different subtypes of intraductal papillary mucinous neoplasm in the pancreas have distinct pathways to pancreatic cancer progression. J Gastroenterol. 2012;47(2):203–13.

Morikawa M, Koinuma D, Miyazono K, Heldin CH. Genome-wide mechanisms of Smad binding. Oncogene. 2012. doi: 10.1038/onc.2012.191.

Ohhashi K, Murakami Y, Maruyama M, Takekoshi T, Ohta H, Ohhashi I, et al. Four cases of mucous secreting pancreatic cancer. (Jpn. Abstr in English). Prog Digest Endosc. 1982;20:348–51.

Samuels Y, Wang Z, Bardelli A, Silliman N, Ptak J, Szabo S, et al. High frequency of mutations of the PIK3CA gene in human cancers. Science. 2004;304(5670):554.

Sasaki S, Yamamoto H, Kaneto H, Ozeki I, Adachi Y, Takagi H, et al. Differential roles of alterations of p53, p16, and SMAD4 expression in the progression of intraductal papillary-mucinous tumors of the pancreas. Oncol Rep. 2003;10(1):21–5.

Satoh K, Shimosegawa T, Moriizumi S, Koizumi M, Toyota T. K-ras mutation and p53 protein accumulation in intraductal mucin-hypersecreting neoplasms of the pancreas. Pancreas. 1996;12(4):362–8.

Schönleben F, Qiu W, Ciau NT, Ho DJ, Li X, Allendorf JD, et al. PIK3CA mutations in intraductal papillary mucinous neoplasm/carcinoma of the pancreas. Clin Cancer Res. 2006;12(12):3851–5.

Serrano M, Hannon GJ, Beach D. A new regulatory motif in cell-cycle control causing specific inhibition of cyclin D/CDK4. Nature. 1993;366(6456):704–7.

Tanaka M, Fernandez-del Castillo C, Adsay V, Chari S, Falconi M, Jang JY, et al. International consensus guidelines 2012 for the management of IPMN and MCN of the pancreas. Pancreatol. 2012;12(3):183–97.

Thatcher JD. The Ras-MAPK signal transduction pathway. Sci Signal. 2010;3(119):tr1.

Wu J, Jiao Y, Dal Molin M, Maitra A, de Wilde RF, Wood LD, et al. Whole-exome sequencing of neoplastic cysts of the pancreas reveals recurrent mutations in components of ubiquitin-dependent pathways. Proc Natl Acad Sci U S A. 2011a;108(52):21188–93.

Wu J, Matthaei H, Maitra A, Dal Molin M, Wood LD, Eshleman JR, et al. Recurrent GNAS mutations define an unexpected pathway for pancreatic cyst development. Sci Transl Med. 2011b; 3(92):92ra66.

Xiao HD, Yamaguchi H, Dias-Santagata D, Kuboki Y, Akhavanfard S, Hatori T, et al. Molecular characteristics and biological behaviours of the oncocytic and pancreatobiliary subtypes of intraductal papillary mucinous neoplasms. J Pathol. 2011;224(4):508–16.

Yamaguchi H, Kuboki Y, Hatori T, Yamamoto M, Shiratori K, Kawamura S, et al. Somatic mutations in PIK3CA and activation of AKT in intraductal tubulopapillary neoplasms of the pancreas. Am J Surg Pathol. 2011;35(12):1812–7.

Yonezawa S, Horinouchi M, Osako M, Kubo M, Takao S, Arimura Y, et al. Gene expression of gastric type mucin (MUC5AC) in pancreatic tumors: its relationship with the biological behavior of the tumor. Pathol Int. 1999;49(1):45–54.

Part II
Investigation

Chapter 5
CT and MRI/MRCP

Kousei Ishigami

Abstract The roles of multidetector-row computed tomography (MDCT) and magnetic resonance imaging (MRI)/MR cholangiopancreatography (MRCP) in the diagnosis of intraductal papillary mucinous neoplasm (IPMN) include the detection, characterization, evaluation of surgical anatomy, and imaging follow-up.

MRI/MRCP is superior to MDCT in the detection and characterization of IPMN. Since branch duct IPMN (BD-IPMN) is relatively common, imaging findings of BD-IPMN may overlap those of other pancreatic cysts. Especially when MDCT or MRI/MRCP fail to demonstrate communication with the main pancreatic duct (MPD), the differential diagnosis between BD-IPMN and oligocystic serous cystic neoplasm (SCN) may be difficult. The likelihood of malignancy has been mainly assessed by indirect findings related to tumor volume and the degree of mucin hypersecretion, including the presence or absence of mural nodule, cyst size, and MPD diameter.

MDCT compensates for the drawbacks of MRI, especially in cases where the image quality is degraded. Due to its higher spatial resolution, MDCT may be helpful in demonstrating pancreatic parenchymal abnormalities indicative of invasive carcinoma. In addition, MDCT is a reliable modality in evaluating preoperative vascular anatomy. Furthermore, curved planar reformation images created along the course of the MPD are visually demonstrable.

MRI/MRCP is the preferred modality for follow-up imaging because of its lacking in ionizing radiation. MDCT is being utilized adjunctively in the imaging surveillance for pancreatic ductal adenocarcinoma (PDAC) and extrapancreatic diseases.

Keywords Characterization of pancreatic cysts • Differential diagnosis of pancreatic cysts • Intraductal papillary mucinous neoplasm (IPMN) • Magnetic resonance cholangiopancreatography (MRCP) • Magnetic resonance imaging (MRI) • Multidetector-row computed tomography (MDCT)

K. Ishigami (✉)
Department of Radiology, University of Iowa Hospitals and Clinics,
Iowa City, IA 52242, USA
e-mail: Ishigamikousei@aol.com

M. Tanaka (ed.), *Intraductal Papillary Mucinous Neoplasm of the Pancreas*,
DOI 10.1007/978-4-431-54472-2_5, © Springer Japan 2014

5.1 The Advantages and Disadvantages of MDCT and MRI/ MRCP

5.1.1 Advantages and Disadvantages of MDCT

The advantages and disadvantages of MDCT are summarized in Table 5.1.

The advantages of MDCT are higher spatial resolution, faster scan time, and wider anatomical coverage. The advancement of MDCT enables us to obtain thin section (≤1 mm) images that have dramatically improved the quality of 3-dimensional (3D) and multiplanar capabilities. Multiplanar reformation (MPR) images of MDCT are useful for lesion detection and image demonstration. Owing to its faster scan time, MDCT has improved the examination throughput even with whole body scans. In addition, faster scan time reduces image degradation by motion (e.g., respiration). The image quality of MDCT is generally consistent in each institution as long as the scan protocol is appropriate. For these reasons, MDCT has been more widely utilized than MRI for the routine clinical purpose in the field of body imaging. Therefore, many physicians feel more comfortable reading.

The administration of intravenous (IV) contrast is necessary for the MDCT evaluation of the pancreas provided there are not any contraindications to IV contrast. Pancreas protocol is the multiphasic study which includes the pancreatic parenchymal (late arterial) and portal venous phases. The pancreatic parenchymal phase corresponds to the peak enhancement of the normal pancreatic parenchyma, during which the contrast (the difference in the Hounsfield units) between pancreatic ductal adenocarcinoma (PDAC) and the normal pancreatic parenchyma is the maximum (McNulty et al. 2001). Pancreas protocol is indicated in cases where the study purpose includes the surveillance for PDAC. Unenhanced CT and the delayed (or equilibrium) phase are optional depending on institutional preference.

The argument in respect to multiphasic study is related to radiation exposure, which is well known but one of the most important disadvantages of MDCT.

Table 5.1 The advantages and disadvantages of MDCT and MRI/MRCP

	Advantage	Disadvantage	Clinical implications
MDCT	Spatial resolution Fast examination time Easy to read for many physicians Wider anatomical coverage	Radiation exposure Time-consuming 3D reconstruction Large volume of data (data explosion) More side effects of IV contrast	Local invasion Vascular anatomy Evaluation of extrapancreatic diseases
MRI	Contrast resolution No radiation exposure Less side effects of IV contrast	Susceptible to artifact Susceptible to image degradation Longer examination time Limited anatomical coverage Higher cost	Detection of pancreatic cysts Characterization of pancreatic cysts Biliary and pancreatic ductal anatomy Imaging follow-up Stone disease

The other disadvantage of MDCT is a limitation of tissue contrast (contrast resolution). For example, pancreatic cysts and MPD dilatation may be obscured if the background pancreatic parenchyma shows fatty infiltration.

5.1.2 Advantages and Disadvantages of MRI/MRCP

The advantages and disadvantages of MRI/MRCP are summarized in Table 5.1.

MRI has higher contrast resolution than MDCT and is very sensitive in depicting free water (i.e., pancreatic cysts, bile duct, and MPD). The prevalence of incidental pancreatic cysts on CT ranged from 1.2 % (Spinelli et al. 2004) to 2.6 % (Laffan et al. 2008) while that of MRI was reported to be 19.9 % (Zhang et al. 2002). The difference reflects the superiority of MRI over MDCT for the detection of pancreatic cysts.

Signal characteristics of MRI (e.g., hemorrhage, proteinaceous fluid, fat, restricted diffusion) may provide additional information to characterize the pancreatic lesions. MRI/MRCP is more sensitive in depicting cyst septations. MRCP can better evaluate the relationship between the MPD and pancreatic cysts (e.g., the communication with MPD). For these reasons, MRI/MRCP can better characterize pancreatic cysts compared to MDCT (Berland et al. 2010; Waters et al. 2008).

There are two types of MRCP sequences: 2D- and 3D-MRCP. 2D-MRCP needs breath-hold. 3D-MRCP is obtained under respiratory gating. 3D-MRCP has higher spatial resolution and signal-to-noise ratio than 2D-MRCP, and it is better in evaluating the detail of pancreatic cyst and duct communication (Yoon et al. 2009) although the source images of 3D-MRCP may appear blurry. Thick slab 2D-MRCP and 3D reconstruction of 3D-MRCP are convenient to overview the pancreaticobiliary ducts. Thin slab 2D-MRCP and source images of MRCP are useful to evaluate the communication with pancreatic duct, mural nodule, septation, and stone disease.

MRI/MRCP is susceptible to artifact. Patient cooperation (e.g., breath hold and steady breathing) is necessary to preserve the image quality. The image quality may differ between different MRI scanners and institutions. The image degradation and artifacts significantly limit image interpretation, which may subsequently cause interobserver disagreement. In addition, it should be emphasized that MRI/MRCP has less spatial resolution than MDCT. Furthermore, longer examination time and higher cost are other disadvantages of MRI/MRCP.

5.2 MDCT and MRI/MRCP Findings of IPMN

5.2.1 Morphologic Subtypes of IPMN

IPMN is a common cystic neoplasm of the pancreas. Imaging findings reflect cystic dilatation of branch and/or main pancreatic ducts owing to mucin hypersecretion. IPMN is classified into three types: branch duct (BD-IPMN), main duct (MD-IPMN), and mixed type (Figs. 5.1, 5.2, 5.3, and 5.4). BD-IPMN is characterized as pancreatic

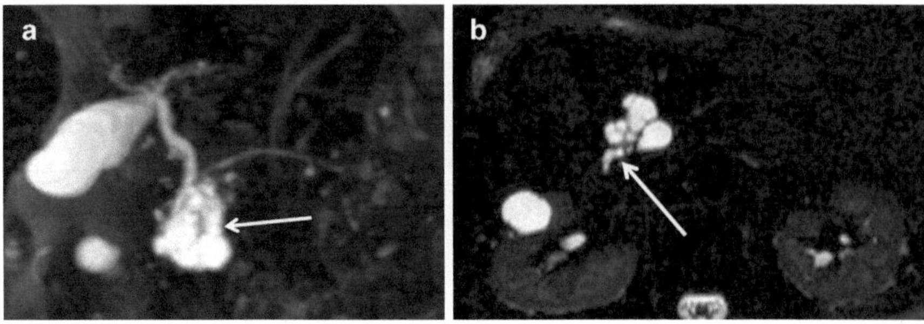

Fig. 5.1 Branch duct-type IPMN (BD-IPMN). The final diagnosis was noninvasive carcinoma. (**a**) Maximum intensity projection (MIP) image of 3D-MRCP shows lobulated multilocular cystic mass in the head of the pancreas (*arrow*). (**b**) Axial MRCP shows the communication with the main pancreatic duct (MPD, *arrow*). No mural nodule is visualized

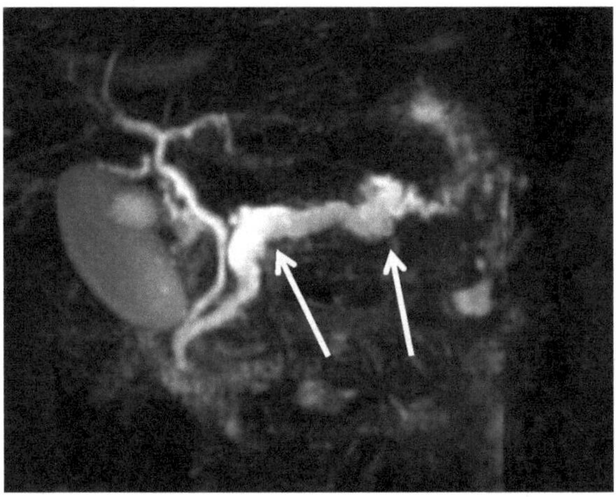

Fig. 5.2 Main duct-type IPMN (MD-IPMN). The final diagnosis was adenoma. MIP image of 3D-MRCP shows cystic dilatation of the MPD (*arrows*) mainly involving the pancreatic body with downstream MPD dilatation

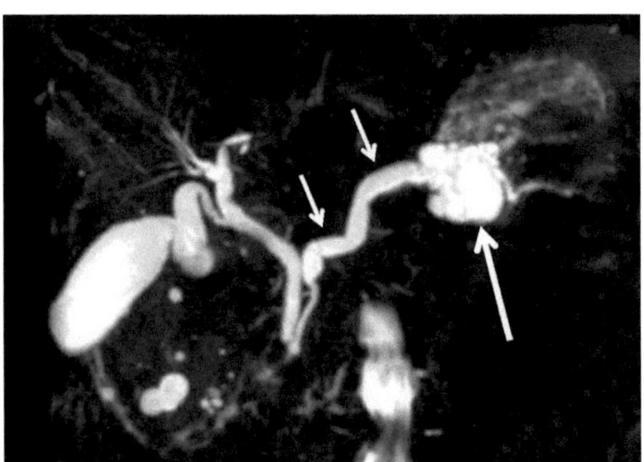

Fig. 5.3 Predominantly BD-IPMN. The final diagnosis was adenoma. Histologically, both branch ducts and the MPD were involved (mixed type). MIP image of 3D-MRCP shows multilocular cystic mass (*large arrow*) with downstream MPD dilatation

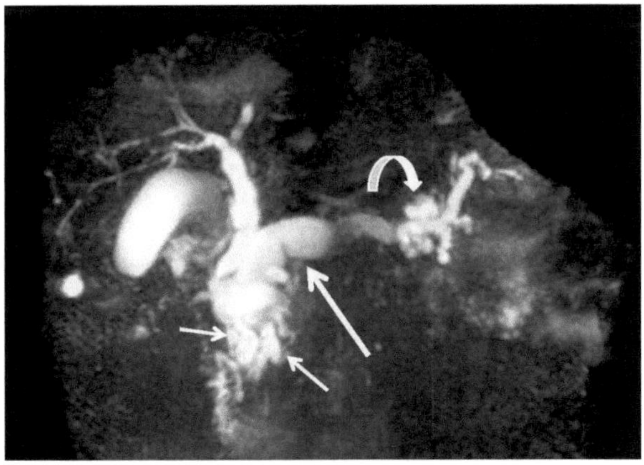

Fig. 5.4 Predominantly MD-IPMN. The final diagnosis was noninvasive carcinoma. Both MPD and branch ducts were involved. MIP image of 3D-MRCP shows cystic dilatation of the MPD in the head and body of the pancreas (*large arrow*) with multiple dilated branch ducts (*small arrows*). Small branch duct IPMNs are also noted in the tail of the pancreas (*curved arrow*)

cysts >5 mm in diameter that communicate with the main pancreatic duct (MPD). MD-IPMN is characterized by segmental or diffuse dilatation of the MPD of >5 mm without other causes of obstruction. Mixed-type IPMN meets the criteria for both BD- and MD-IPMN (Tanaka et al. 2012). BD-IPMN is occasionally multifocal. Multiplicity of IPMN may influence preoperative strategy and postoperative follow-up planning (Tanaka et al. 2012; Mori et al. 2012). The multiplicity of IPMN is more suitable to be evaluated by MRI/MRCP because MRI is more sensitive in detecting small pancreatic cysts.

5.2.2 *Branch Duct IPMN (BD-IPMN)*

BD-IPMN presents as a multilocular or unilocular cystic mass. BD-IPMN represents a cluster of dilated branch ducts, which is typically lobulated in shape ("grape-like" shape). The thickness and contrast enhancement of cyst wall is variable. The cyst wall may be thin or thick depending on coexisting inflammation or tumor infiltration (Fig. 5.5). The key for the diagnosis of BD-IPMN is the communication with the MPD. Downstream MPD is typically dilated or prominent. If these findings are clear, the diagnosis of BD-IPMN is not difficult. However, even in a relatively larger MD-IPMN (>3 cm), MDCT and MRCP may fail to demonstrate communication with the MPD (Figs. 5.5 and 5.6). In such cases, the differential diagnosis is problematic because imaging findings may overlap those of other cystic lesions of the pancreas.

5.3 Differential Diagnoses of BD-IPMN

Differential diagnoses of BD-IPMN are summarized in Table 5.2.

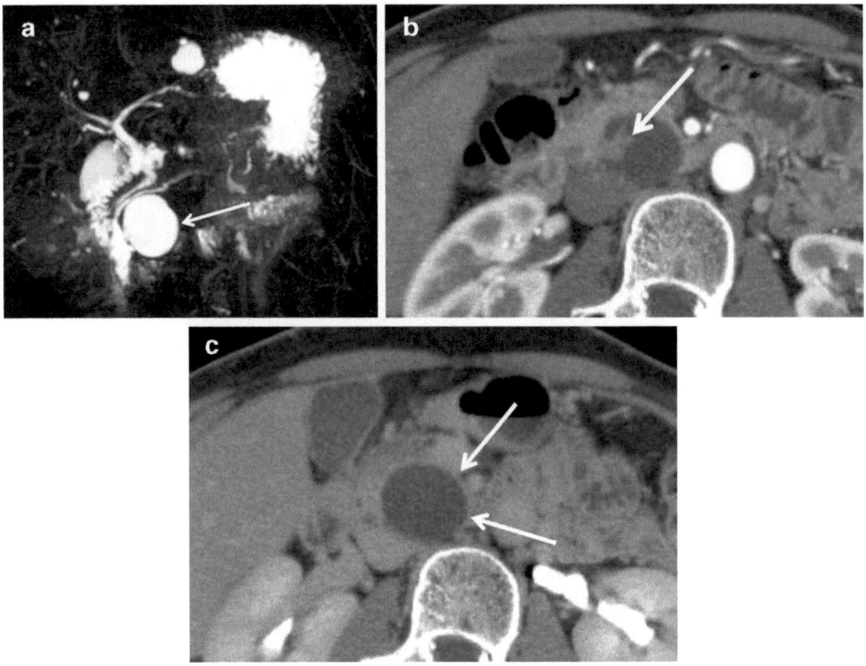

Fig. 5.5 BD-IPMN with wall enhancement and mural nodule. In this case, MRCP and MDCT were unable to demonstrate the communication with MPD. The presence of wall enhancement is not typical for a macrocyst of serous cystic neoplasm (SCN). The location (pancreatic head) is not typical for mucinous cystic neoplasm. The final diagnosis was noninvasive carcinoma. Noninvasive carcinoma was found in the mural nodule and cyst wall. (**a**) MIP image of 3D-MRCP demonstrates unilocular cystic mass in the head of the pancreas (*arrow*). However, the communication with the MPD is unclear. (**b**) Pancreatic parenchymal phase of axial MDCT shows a papillary mural nodule (*arrow*). (**c**) The equilibrium (delayed) phase of axial MDCT shows enhancing cyst wall (*arrows*)

5.3.1 Serous Cystic Neoplasm (SCN)

Pancreatic serous cystic neoplasm (SCN) is almost always benign (98.8 %) (Kimura et al. 2012). Differentiating between BD-IPMN and SCN is important. SCN is classified into microcystic, oligocystic, solid variant, and mixed types. Microcystic type consists of a cluster of microcyst, which is the so-called honeycomb pattern (Choi et al. 2009). Macrocyst is defined as a cyst measuring more than 2 cm (or 1 cm) in diameter. Wall of macrocyst is thin and wall enhancement is not typically seen (Yamaguchi et al. 2007). Oligocystic type consists of a macrocyst and a few small cysts, showing "cyst-by-cyst" pattern. Solid variant (solid serous adenoma) is extremely rare. Even though imaging findings often appear solid, it may be histologically microcystic. Mixed type is a combination of two or more different components, most commonly consisting of microcystic and macrocystic components. Typically, microcysts are noted in the center, and macrocyst and relatively larger

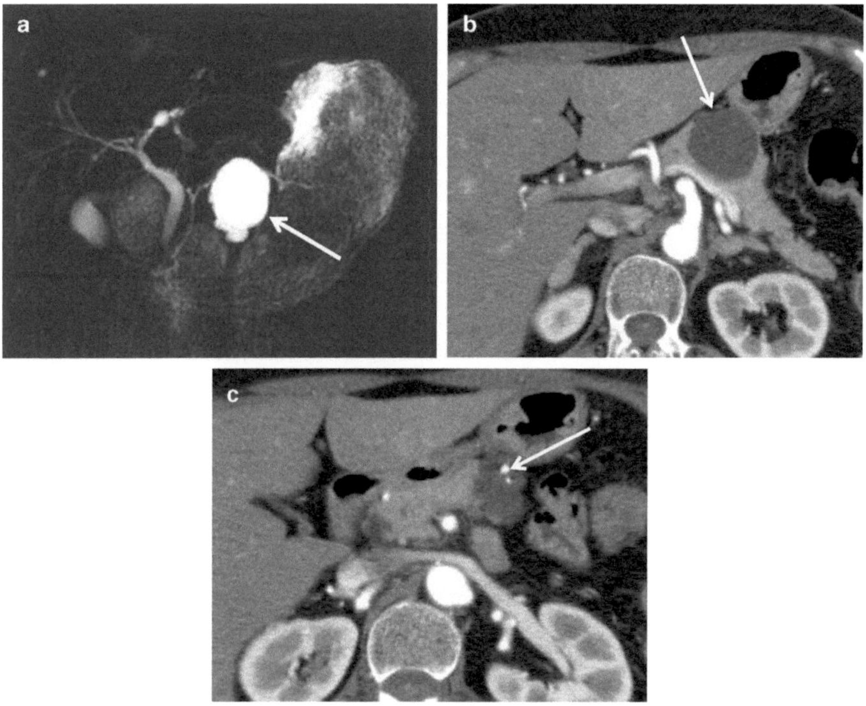

Fig. 5.6 BD-IPMN mimicking oligocystic serous cystic neoplasm (SCN). The final diagnosis was adenoma. (**a**) Thick slab 2D-MRCP shows a lobulated cystic mass in the body of the pancreas (*arrow*). Source image and thin slab MRCP fail to demonstrate communication with the MPD (not shown). The morphology of the cystic lesion mimics oligocystic SCN, showing cyst-by-cyst pattern (see Fig. 5.8). (**b**, **c**) The pancreatic parenchymal phase of axial MDCT shows a thin-walled cyst (**b**) with calcification (**c**) (*arrows*)

cysts are located peripherally. However, honeycomb pattern may be seen peripherally (Fig. 5.7). The key for the diagnosis of SCN is to look for honeycomb pattern. On the other hand, distinguishing oligocystic SCN from BD-IPMN may be difficult on MDCT or MRI/MRCP because a cluster of microcysts is not recognized in oligocystic SCN (Fig. 5.8). In such cases, ERCP (to evaluate the communication with the MPD) or EUS-guided fluid aspiration may be necessary for further characterization. In addition, some microcystic SCN may be erroneously characterized as BD-IPMN with mural nodule because fibrosis in SCN may mimic mural nodule (Choi et al. 2009) (Fig. 5.9).

5.3.2 *Mucinous Cystic Neoplasm (MCN)*

Mucinous cystic neoplasm (MCN) is almost always located in the pancreatic body/tail (99.4 %) in female patients (98.1 %) (Yamao et al. 2011). The location of the

Table 5.2 Differential diagnoses of BD-IPMN

	Typical morphology	Connection to the MPD	Wall enhancement	Diagnostic pitfall (additional comments)
BD-IPMN	Grape-like	(+) Prominent downstream MPD	(±) Caused by inflammation or tumor infiltration	MDCT/MRCP may fail to demonstrate the communication with the MPD May present with various morphology
SCN	Honeycomb pattern Microcystic	(−)	(−) Macrocystic	Oligocystic SCN without honeycomb pattern may mimic BD-IPMN Fibrosis may mimic mural nodule of IPMN Honeycomb pattern may not always be seen in the center
MCN	Orange-like common capsule	(−) on MRCP/ MDCT	(+)	Cyst wall may not always be thick (Extremely rare for male) (Extremely rare in the pancreatic head)
Retention cyst	Similar to BD-IPMN	(+) Downstream stricture	(±) Caused by inflammation	Pancreatic ductal adenocarcinoma Difficult to evaluate branch duct stricture

lesion and the patient's sex are very important for the differential diagnosis. The communication with the MPD was reported to be 18.1 % of MCN (Yamao et al. 2011) although the communication with the MPD is not clearly demonstrated by MDCT or MRI/MRCP. Owing to the presence of a common capsule, it is well known that the shape of MCN is called "orange-like." However, some BD-IPMN may morphologically mimic MCN, and cyst wall thickening or wall enhancement is not helpful for the differential diagnosis (Fig. 5.10). Both IPMN and MCN have malignant potential. In general, surgical resection is indicated for MCN. However, it has been reported that MCNs less than 4 cm in diameter without mural nodule were benign (Reddy et al. 2004; Crippa et al. 2008).

5.3.3 Other Differential Diagnoses of BD-IPMN

Retention cyst may show similar imaging appearance to BD-IPMN because retention cyst reflects dilatation of branch ducts and/or MPD (Fig. 5.11). The presence or absence of stricture of the downstream pancreatic duct is the key to distinguishing retention cyst from BD-IPMN. For retention cyst, the cause of pancreatic ductal stricture should be further evaluated to exclude PDAC. Although it is uncommon,

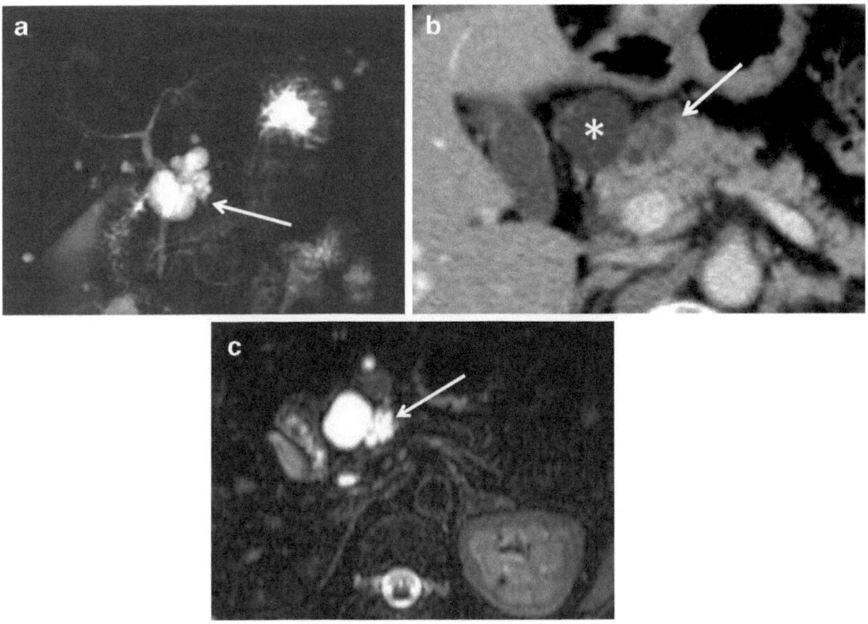

Fig. 5.7 Mixed-type serous cystic neoplasm (mixed microcystic and macrocystic SCN). (**a**) Thick slab 2D-MRCP demonstrates a lobulated multilocular cystic mass in the pancreatic head (*arrow*). (**b**) The portal venous phase of axial MDCT shows thin-walled macrocyst (*asterisk*) and cluster of microcysts (*arrow*). (**c**) Axial thin slab MRCP more clearly shows a cluster of microcysts (*honey-comb pattern*, *arrow*). MRI better characterizes this cystic lesion than MDCT

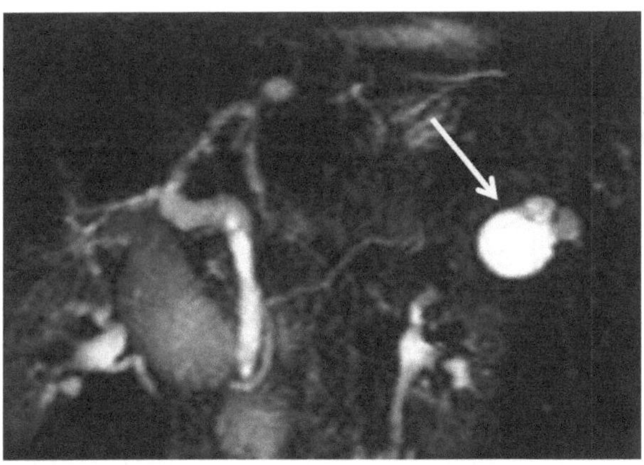

Fig. 5.8 Oligocystic SCN. Thick slab MRCP shows a lobulated multilocular cystic mass, showing cyst-by-cyst pattern (*arrow*)

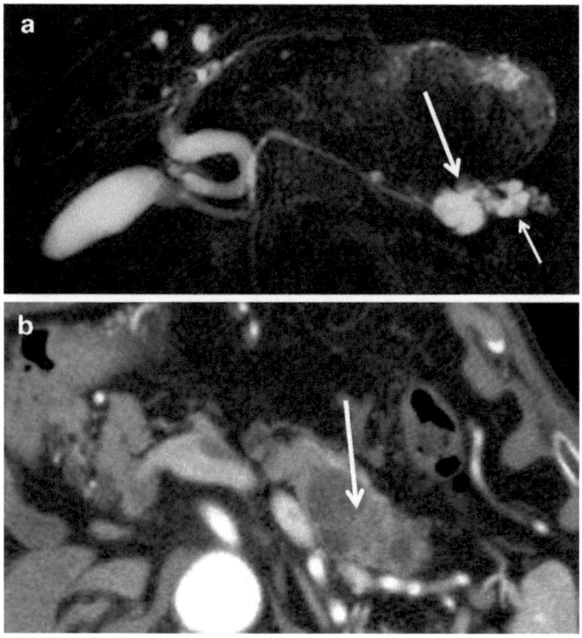

Fig. 5.9 Microcystic SCN mimicking IPMN with mural nodule. (**a**) Thick slab 2D-MRCP shows multilocular cystic mass in the pancreatic tail (*large arrow*). The upstream site simulates dilatation of the MPD (*small arrow*). ERCP (not shown) was unremarkable without MPD dilatation or opacification of the cyst. (**b**) The pancreatic parenchymal phase of axial contrast-enhanced MDCT demonstrates an enhancing area in the cystic lesion, mimicking mural nodule (*arrow*). The enhancing area turned out to represent fibrosis

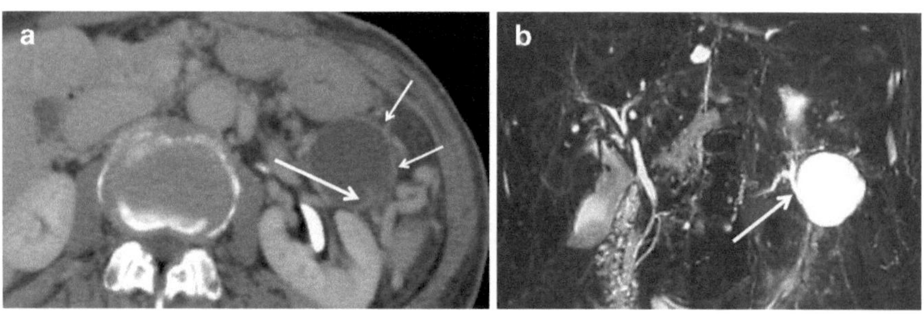

Fig. 5.10 BD-IPMN mimicking mucinous cystic neoplasm (MCN). The final diagnosis was noninvasive carcinoma. Although the mural nodule represented adenoma, noninvasive carcinoma was found in the cyst wall. (**a**) The equilibrium phase of contrast-enhanced axial MDCT shows cystic mass with mural nodule (*large arrow*) and cyst wall enhancement (*small arrows*). (**b**) 3D-MRCP shows a dilated branch duct connecting with the cystic lesion (*arrow*), favoring the diagnosis of BD-IPMN rather than MCN

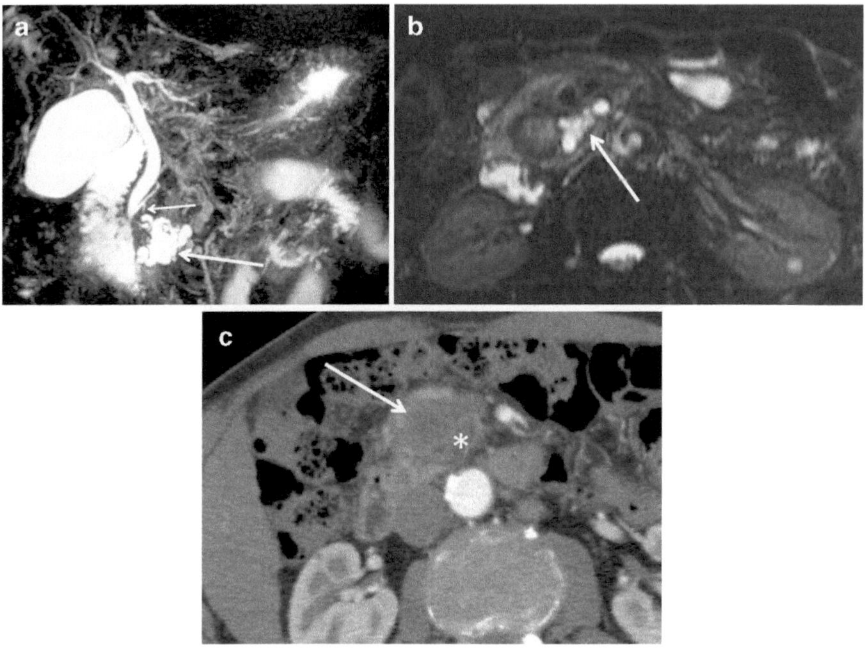

Fig. 5.11 Retention cyst mimicking BD-IPMN caused by pancreatic head ductal adenocarcinoma (PDAC). (**a**) 3D-MRCP shows a multilocular cystic lesion in the pancreatic head (*large arrow*). The shape of this cystic lesion is similar to BD-IPMN. Narrowing of the branch duct is suspected (*small arrow*) although it is indeterminate considering the limited spatial resolution of MRCP. (**b**) Axial MRCP demonstrates the cystic lesion to represent dilated branch ducts in the uncinate process (*arrow*). (**c**) The pancreatic parenchymal phase shows a hypoattenuating solid mass in the pancreatic head (*arrow*), consistent with PDAC. The cystic lesion (*asterisk*) turned out to be a retention cyst caused by the presence of PDAC and resultant stricture of the uncinate branch duct. On MDCT, the retention cyst is inconspicuous because of the poor contrast to adjacent PDAC (see Fig. 5.11b)

BD-IPMN with large or multiple mural nodules may mimic solid pancreatic tumors (Fig. 5.12) with necrosis/degeneration such as neuroendocrine tumor and solid pseudopapillary neoplasm.

5.3.4 Main Duct IPMN (MD-IPMN) and Differential Diagnoses

MD-IPMN is characterized as diffuse or focal dilatation of the MPD without downstream MPD stricture. The MPD diameter of 5 mm or more is reported to be a sensitive diagnostic criterion (Tanaka et al. 2012). Differential diagnosis of MD-IPMN includes chronic pancreatitis. Both MD-IPMN and chronic pancreatitis may show

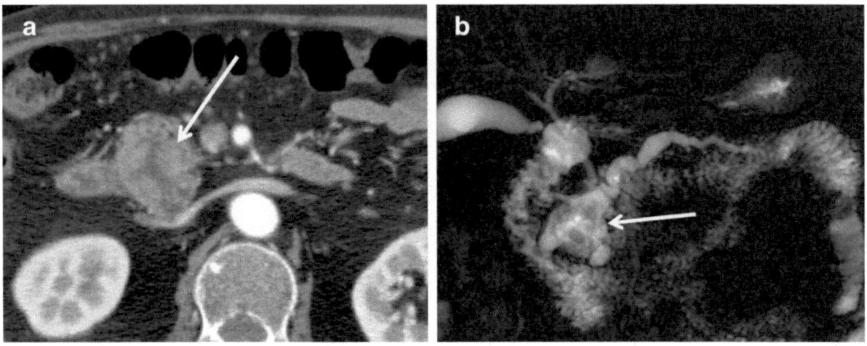

Fig. 5.12 Mixed-type IPMN mimicking solid tumor on MDCT. The final diagnosis was noninvasive carcinoma. (**a**) The pancreatic parenchymal phase of axial MDCT shows an enhancing tumor in the pancreatic head (*arrow*) with upstream MPD dilatation (not shown). (**b**) Thick slab 2D-MRCP clearly demonstrates the tumor to be confined in the main and branch pancreatic ducts. In this case, it was difficult to classify whether it was predominantly MD-IPMN or BD-IPMN (mixed type)

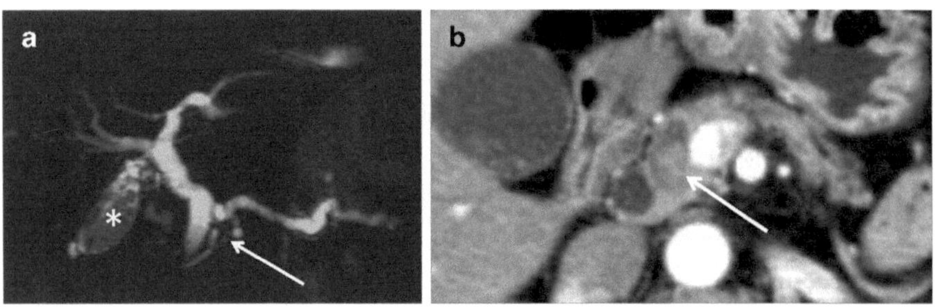

Fig. 5.13 IPMN without mucin hypersecretion. The final diagnosis was invasive carcinoma. (**a**) Thick slab 2D-MRCP shows filling defect in the MPD in the pancreatic head (*arrow*) with upstream MPD dilatation. There is no downstream MPD dilatation. Multiple gallbladder stones are noted (*asterisk*). (**b**) The pancreatic parenchymal phase of axial MDCT shows enhancing mass (*arrow*) that corresponds to the filling defect noted on MRCP

marked atrophy of the pancreatic parenchyma (Pedrosa and Boparai 2010). IPMN without mucin hypersecretion is an unusual form of IPMN (Fig. 5.13). IPMN without mucin hypersecretion presents as an intraluminal mass in the MPD (and/or a branch duct) without downstream MPD dilatation. Other intraductal pancreatic tumors such as intraductal tubulopapillary neoplasm and ductal invasion from hypovascular neuroendocrine tumor or acinar cell carcinoma may show similar imaging findings (Yamaguchi et al. 2009; Ishigami et al. 2008) (Fig. 5.14).

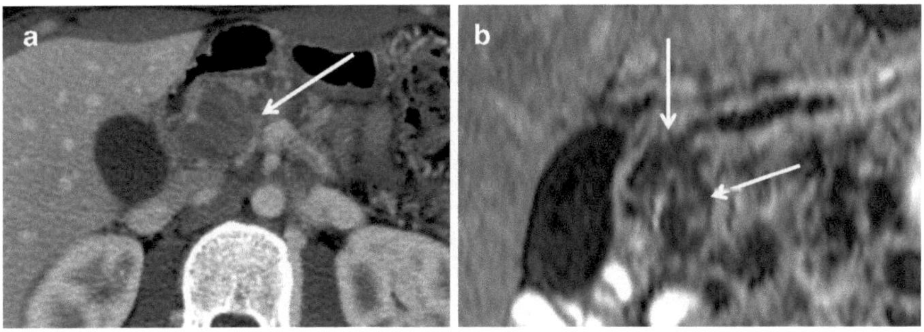

Fig. 5.14 Acinar cell carcinoma growing in the pancreatic duct. (**a**) The portal venous phase of axial MDCT shows hypoattenuating mass in the pancreatic head (*arrow*). (**b**) Post-contrast curved planar reformatted image of dynamic MRI demonstrates the tumor to be confined in the main pancreatic and branch ducts (*arrows*)

5.4 MDCT and MRI/MRCP Evaluations of IPMN Characterization of IPMN in Table 5.3

5.4.1 Likelihood of Malignancy

The radiological prediction of malignancy in IPMN is challenging. It is based on indirect findings including the presence or absence of mural nodule, cyst size (BD-IPMN), and MPD diameter. These parameters reflect the tumor volume and the degree of mucin hypersecretion. Namely, as the tumor volume and the degree of mucin hypersecretion increase, the likelihood of malignancy also increases.

5.4.2 Radiological Classification of Morphologic Subtypes of IPMN

The frequency of malignancy is different for each morphologic subtype. The frequencies of malignancy were 62.2 % (43.6 % for invasive carcinoma) in MD-IPMN, 24.4 % (16.6 %) in BD-IPMN, and 57.6 % (45.3 %) in mixed type (Tanaka et al. 2012). The classification of the morphological subtypes is important for clinical management although the definition of mixed-type IPMN may vary. In preoperative imaging studies, it is desirable to classify as MD-IPMN or BD-IPMN based on the predominant pattern of ductal dilatation (Figs. 5.3 and 5.4).

5.4.3 MPD Diameter

The frequency of malignant IPMN is similar between MD-IPMN and mixed-type IPMN, which indicates the involvement of the MPD is higher frequency of malignancy.

Table 5.3 Comparison of international consensus guidelines 2012 for the management of IPMN and MCN of the pancreas (Tanaka et al. 2012) and flow chart for an asymptomatic patient with an incidental pancreatic cystic mass by the American College of Radiology (Berland et al. 2010)

	International consensus guidelines 2012	American College of Radiology
BD-IPMN or cyst <1 cm	Follow-up by CT/MRI in 2–3 years	Single follow-up 1 year preferably by MRI
BD-IPMN or cyst <2 cm	Follow-up by CT/MRI yearly times 2 years, then lengthen interval if no change	If stable, no further work-up If growth, imaging characterization preferably by MRI/MRCP (see BD-IPMN 2–3 cm)
BD-IPMN 2–3 cm	EUS in 3–6 months, then lengthen interval alternating MRI with EUS as appropriate Consider surgery in young, fit patients with need for prolonged surveillance	Follow-up every 6 months for 2 years If no growth after 2 years, follow up yearly If growth or suspicious features develop, consider resection
BD-IPMN >3 cm	Close surveillance alternating MRI with EUS every 3–6 months Strongly consider surgery in young, fit patients with need for prolonged surveillance	Cyst aspiration Resect, depending on comorbidities and risk

Note. The table only refers to BD-IPMN without worrisome features or high-risk stigmata (e.g., mural nodule, MPD dilatation) according to the international consensus guidelines 2012. The American College of Radiology (ACR) only includes asymptomatic and incidental pancreatic cyst. The American College of Radiology does not describe the characterization of a pancreatic cyst <2 cm, which may or may not include BD-IPMN <2 cm

The MPD involvement reflects the degree of MPD dilatation. The measurement of the MPD is usually given by the maximum diameter. Diffuse dilatation of the MPD predicts a higher probability of malignancy than focal or segmental dilatation (Manfredi et al. 2009; Irie et al. 2000). Manfredi et al. (2009) described that the mean diameter of MPD in malignant IPMN (18 mm) was larger than benign IPMN (11 mm). In addition, wall enhancement of the MPD was more frequently observed in malignant IPMN (74 %) than benign IPMN (21 %) (Manfredi et al. 2009). However, wall enhancement of the MPD may be seen secondary to inflammation. Kawamoto et al. (2006) described that the MPD caliber is larger in patients with invasive carcinoma (9.3 ± 5.5 mm) than those with noninvasive carcinoma and adenoma (4.6 ± 4.1 mm). Ogawa et al. described that the invasiveness of IPMN significantly increased as the maximum diameter of the MPD increased: the mean diameters of the MPD were 5.8 ± 3.7 mm, 11.0 ± 6.6 mm, and 14.7 ± 8.2 mm in adenoma, noninvasive carcinoma, and invasive carcinoma, respectively, and the MPD diameter of 6 mm or more was one of the significant predictors of malignancy (Ogawa et al. 2008). On the other hand, Gupta et al. (2008) described that it was difficult to diagnose invasive carcinoma based on the MPD diameter [adenoma (4.5 ± 4.3 mm), noninvasive carcinoma (11.9 ± 15.9 mm), and invasive carcinoma (13.9 ± 10.9 mm)]. Dilatation of the MPD suggests higher likelihood of malignancy.

However, the caliber of the MPD may overlap among adenoma, noninvasive carcinoma, and invasive carcinoma. International consensus guidelines 2012 for the management of IPMN and MCN of the pancreas described that the MPD diameters of 5–9 mm and ≥10 mm are a worrisome feature and high-risk stigma for malignant IPMN, respectively (Tanaka et al. 2012).

5.4.4 Cyst Size

The largest diameter is measured for the cyst size of BD-IPMN. When utilizing MDCT, it is recommended to utilize MPR images to avoid underestimation of the cyst size. For BD-IPMN, diameter of more than 3 cm (Sugiyama et al. 2003) or 4 cm (Nara et al. 2009) has been correlated with malignancy, and the international consensus guidelines set 3 cm in diameter as a threshold for worrisome feature of malignancy (Tanaka et al. 2012). However, cyst size may be a weak predictor for malignancy (Tanaka et al. 2012; Irie et al. 2000). Thick enhancing cyst wall and/or septae, irregularity of the cyst wall, and a wide (>1 cm) connection with the MPD were other findings that can suggest malignancy (Pedrosa and Boparai 2010; Gupta et al. 2008; Nara et al. 2009) although cyst wall enhancement may be seen secondary to inflammation.

5.4.5 Mural Nodule

The presence of mural nodule is one of the most important findings to predict malignancy. MRI/MRCP detected mural nodules in 59 % of patients with malignant IPMN and 4 % of patients with benign IPMN (Manfredi et al. 2009). However, the absence of mural nodule does not preclude malignancy (Fig. 5.1). In addition, the presence of mural nodule is not direct evidence of malignancy because mural nodule may be seen in benign IPMN (Figs. 5.15 and 5.16). Furthermore, the portion of mural nodule may be different from that of carcinoma (Figs. 5.10 and 5.17). Therefore, the presence of mural nodule is an indirect finding that increases the likelihood of malignancy. As the diameter of a mural nodule increases, the likelihood of malignancy and invasiveness increases. However, the size criteria of mural nodule vary in literature, ranging from 3 mm (Sugiyama et al. 2003) to 10 mm (Yamaguchi et al. 1996). Ogawa et al. (2008) found that the largest diameter of a mural nodule in the MPD measuring >3 mm and >6 mm suggested malignant IPMN and invasive carcinoma, respectively. According to Ogawa et al. (2008), same tendency was observed in respect to a mural nodule in BD-IPMN although there were no significant differences.

The detectability of mural nodule by MDCT and MRI/MRCP is grossly similar. The combination of the source images of 3D-MRCP or thin slab 2D-MRCP and contrast-enhanced MRI would be more convincing to evaluate the presence of mural

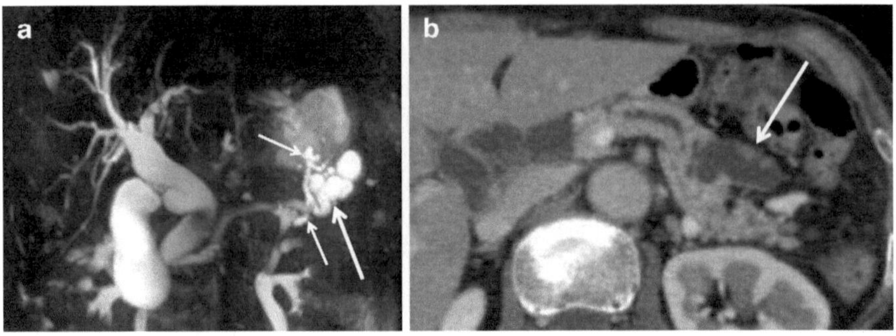

Fig. 5.15 BD-IPMN with mural nodule. The final diagnosis was benign (adenoma). (**a**) MIP image of 3D-MRCP demonstrates a multilocular cystic mass in the border of the pancreatic body and tail with connection to the main pancreatic duct (*large arrow*, MPD). Small BD-IPMNs are also noted (*small arrows*). The extrahepatic bile duct is dilated without bile duct stricture, possible caused by a large periampullary diverticulum (not shown). (**b**) The portal venous of axial MDCT shows an enhancing mural nodule (*arrow*)

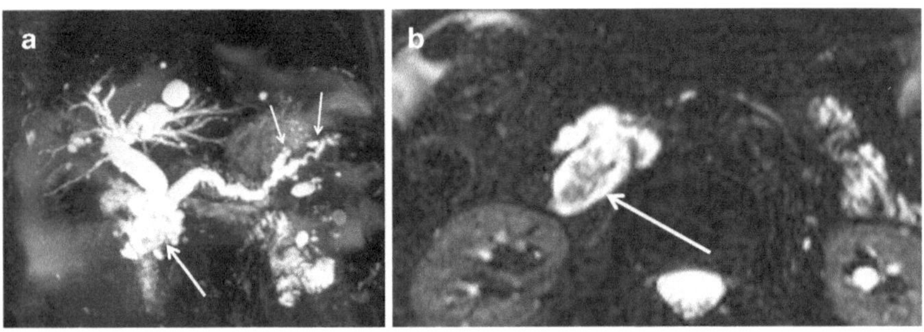

Fig. 5.16 Predominantly MD-IPMN with a large mural nodule in the MPD. The final diagnosis was benign (adenoma). (**a**) MIP image of 3D-MRCP shows dilatation of the MPD and branch ducts mainly in the pancreatic head (*large arrow*). Small BD-IPMNs are also noted (*small arrows*). (**b**) Axial MRCP shows a large mural nodule in the dilated MPD (*arrow*)

nodule. Mural nodule shows either gradual or early enhancement. It is unlikely that the shape or enhancement pattern of mural nodule is predictive for malignancy. In cases where the size of mural nodule is small (<3 or 5 mm), the imaging interpretation may differ between observer. In addition, a small mural nodule is occasionally difficult to correlate with pathological specimen. Such false positive result or discrepancy may be related to the intervening pancreatic tissue, fibrosis or edema, and shrinkage after formalin fixation. Therefore, a small mural nodule without measurable enhancement should be considered a questionable finding.

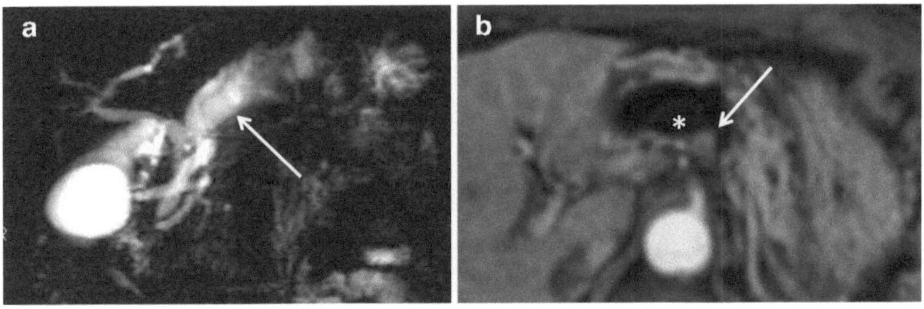

Fig. 5.17 Predominantly MD-IPMN with mural nodule. The final diagnosis was invasive carcinoma. However, invasive carcinoma (microscopic invasion) was found in a dilated branch duct separate from main duct lesion and the mural nodule (adenoma). (**a**) MIP image of 2D-MRCP shows marked dilatation of the MPD in the body and head of the pancreas (*arrow*), consistent with MD-IPMN. (**b**) The portal venous phase of axial dynamic MRI shows an enhancing mural nodule in the MPD (*arrow*) with surrounding mucin pool (*asterisk*)

5.5 Invasive Carcinoma Derived from IPMN and Pancreatic Ductal Adenocarcinoma (PDAC) Concomitant with IPMN

The radiological diagnosis of invasive carcinoma derived from IPMN is possible in cases where the solid lesion in the pancreatic parenchyma can be recognized (Ogawa et al. 2008; Nara et al. 2009; Vullierme et al. 2007) (Fig. 5.18). Associated ductal obstruction is occasionally seen. Delayed enhancement of solid lesion may represent desmoplastic change of invasive carcinoma (Ogawa et al. 2008). Radiological diagnosis of microscopic invasive carcinoma is difficult because there is no direct finding to suggest invasiveness as described previously.

Pancreatic ductal adenocarcinoma (PDAC) concomitant with IPMN is seen 4.1 % of surgically resected IPMN (Yamaguchi et al. 2011) (Fig. 5.19). PDAC concomitant with IPMN is diagnosed based on topologic relationship. Yamaguchi et al. (2011) described that 3.9 % of surgically resected IPMN also had PDAC undetermined relationship with IPMN. Therefore, it is important to pay attention to the presence of PDAC in patients with IPMN.

The diagnostic ability of MDCT and MRI is grossly similar in the diagnosis of PDAC. The modality of choice depends on the institutional preferences. However, MDCT is more familiar to read for many physicians and plays the role of the initial screening for the detection of a smaller PDAC. A small PDAC tends to show iso-attenuation in the pancreatic parenchymal phase (Yoon et al. 2011; Ishigami et al. 2009). In such case, delayed enhancement related to desmoplastic change may be helpful to recognize the lesion (Ishigami et al. 2009). In addition, MRI or PET/CT may be useful for the problem-solving if MDCT findings are equivocal.

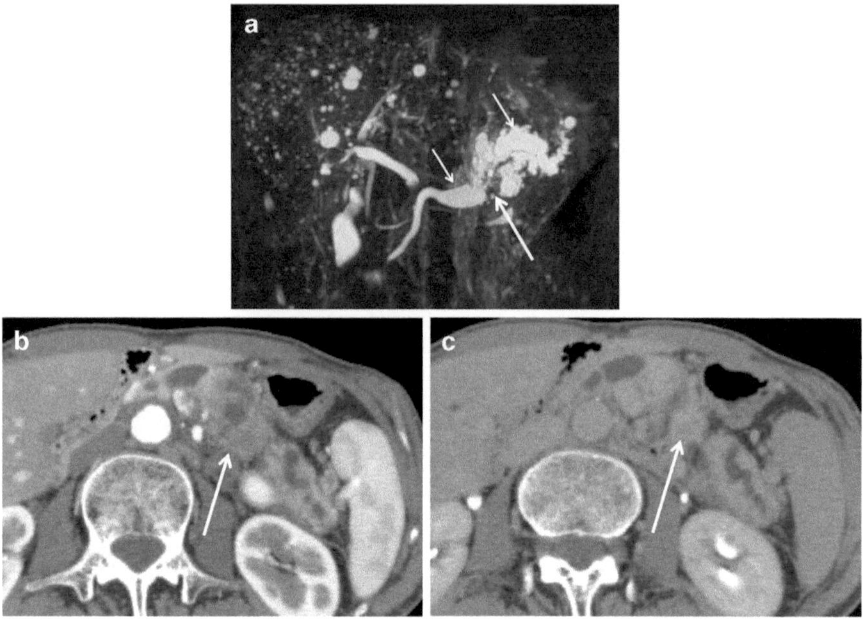

Fig. 5.18 Invasive carcinoma derived from IPMN. (**a**) MIP image of 3D-MRCP demonstrates dilatation of the MPD (*small arrows*) and branch ducts. Solid lesion with narrowing of the MPD is noted (*large arrow*). Multiple cysts and/or biliary hamartomata are seen in the liver. (**b**) The pancreatic parenchymal phase of axial MDCT demonstrates a hypoattenuating solid lesion in the pancreatic parenchyma extending to the peripancreatic fat (*arrow*). (**c**) The equilibrium (delayed) phase of axial MDCT shows delayed enhancement of solid lesion, representing desmoplastic change (*arrow*)

5.6 Preoperative Evaluation of IPMN

Both MRI/MRCP and MDCT are necessary for preoperative evaluation. MDCT is suitable for evaluating local invasion and variant vascular anatomy. However, it has been reported that vascular invasion tended to be overestimated in IPMN due to inflammation (Vullierme et al. 2007).

Additionally, the wider anatomical coverage of MDCT is useful to evaluate not only distant metastasis but also other extrapancreatic diseases. Furthermore, curved planar reformation (CPR) image created along the course of the MPD has visual impact to demonstrate the lesion (Figs. 5.20, 5.21, and 5.22). CPR image may be helpful for postoperative pathology mapping.

5.7 Imaging Follow-Up

MRI/MRCP is preferable for imaging follow-up of IPMN because of its lack of ionizing radiation. However, the image quality influences the modality of choice for imaging follow-up. For example, in patients with status post-pancreaticoduodenectomy,

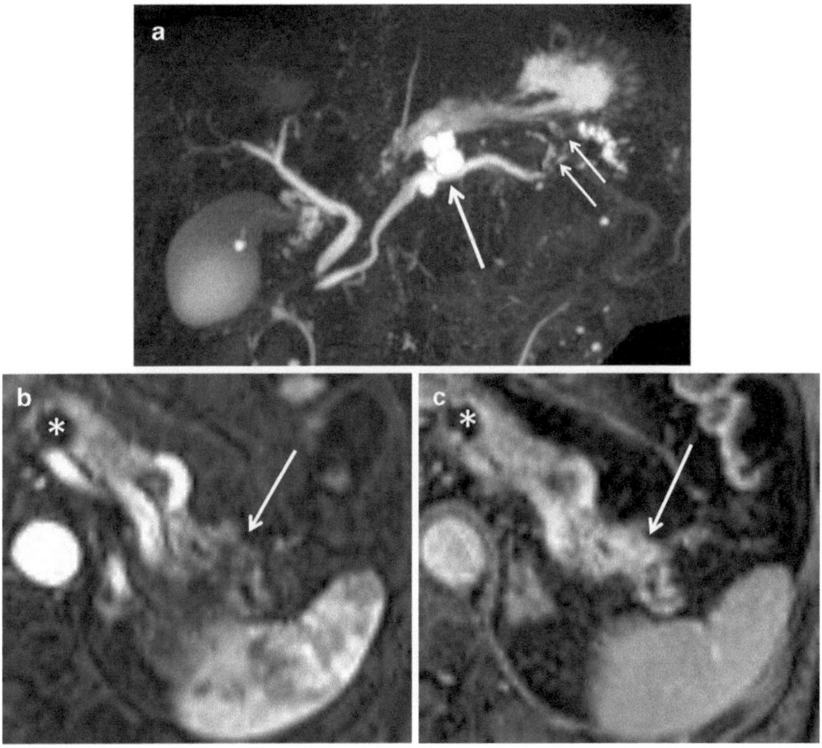

Fig. 5.19 Pancreatic ductal adenocarcinoma in the pancreatic tail with concomitant BD-IPMN (adenoma) in the pancreatic body. (**a**) MIP image of 3D-MRCP shows BD-IPMN in the pancreatic body (*large arrow*). Additionally, obstruction of the MPD and upstream MPD dilatation are noted (*small arrows*). (**b**) The arterial phase of axial dynamic MRI shows a hypointense lesion (*arrow*) in the pancreatic tail that corresponds to the area of MPD obstruction noted on MRCP. *Asterisk* indicates BD-IPMN. (**c**) The equilibrium (delayed) phase of axial dynamic MRI demonstrates the pancreatic tail lesion to show delayed enhancement, consistent with pancreatic cancer (*arrow*). *Asterisk* indicates BD-IPMN

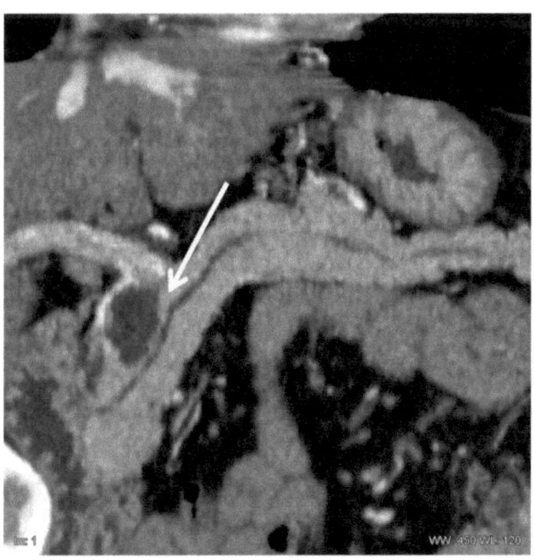

Fig. 5.20 BD-IPMN in the pancreatic head (*arrow*) demonstrated by curved planar reformation (CPR) image created along the course of the MPD (Courtesy of Daisuke Kakihara, M.D., Department of Clinical Radiology, Kyushu University, Fukuoka, Japan)

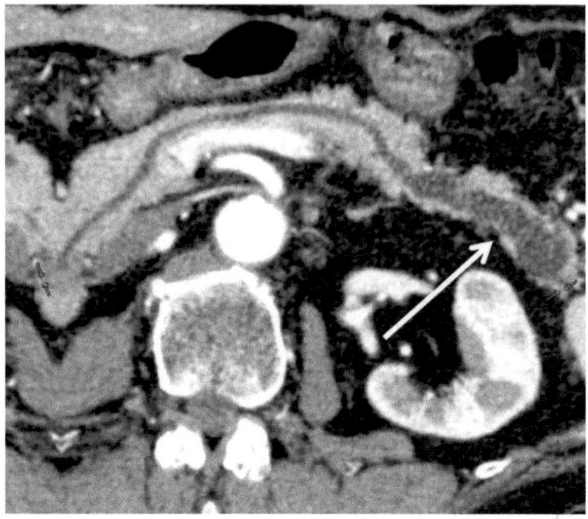

Fig. 5.21 MD-IPMN demonstrated by CPR image, showing segmental dilatation of the MPD in the pancreatic tail (*arrow*) (Courtesy of Hiroyuki Irie, M.D., Department of Radiology, Saga University, Saga, Japan)

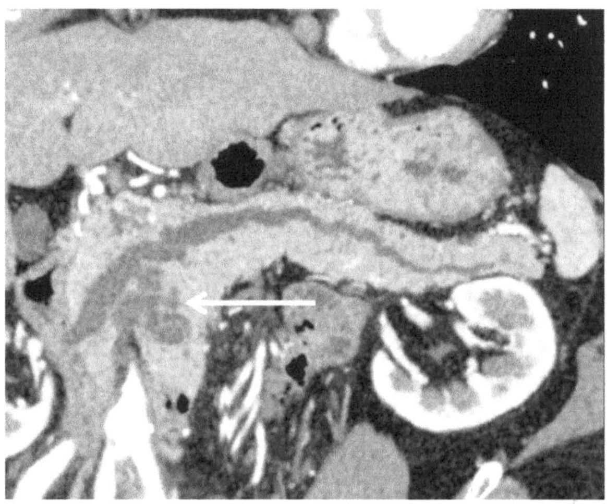

Fig. 5.22 Predominantly BD-IPMN (*arrow*) in the pancreatic head with MPD dilatation demonstrated by CPR image (Courtesy of Hiroyuki Irie, M.D., Department of Radiology, Saga University, Saga, Japan)

the residual pancreas is atrophic, which may limit the evaluation of the pancreatic parenchymal abnormality such as the development of PDAC. In such cases, MDCT should be considered to compensate for the limitations of MRI. In addition, it is easier to evaluate postoperative anatomy on MDCT than on MRI.

The American College of Radiology (ACR) (Berland et al. 2010) recommends BD-IPMN measuring 2–3 cm to be followed up every 6 months for 2 years. If there is no growth after 2 years, interval follow-up can be performed yearly. ACR suggests a pancreatic cyst <2 cm to be followed up in 1 year. If it is stable, no further follow-up is recommended. In addition, cyst aspiration is recommended for pancreatic cysts >3 cm.

In contrast, international consensus guidelines 2012 for the management of IPMN and MCN of the pancreas (Tanaka et al. 2012) recommends more frequent imaging follow-up for BD-IPMN (Table 5.3). Although ACR did not specifically describe imaging management for BD-IPMN <2 cm, many of BD-IPMN <2 cm without mural nodule or MPD dilatation would be included in the category of an asymptomatic patient with an incidental pancreatic cyst <2 cm. Additionally, the majority of BD-IPMN <2 cm without mural nodule or MPD dilatation is expected to be stable after 1-year follow-up (Irie et al. 2004). Therefore, BD-IPMN <2 cm may be lost to be followed up. It is still controversial whether surveillance can be safely spaced or discontinued after long-term stability. Not only interval growth of BD-IPMN but also the possible risk of the development of PDAC should be considered for imaging follow-up of IPMN.

References

Berland LL, Silverman SG, Gore RM, Mayo-Smith WW, Megibow AJ, Yee J, et al. Managing incidental findings on abdominal CT: white paper of the ACR incidental findings committee. J Am Coll Radiol. 2010;7(10):754–73.

Choi JY, Kim MJ, Lee JY, Lim JS, Chung JJ, Kim KW, et al. Typical and atypical manifestations of serous cystadenoma of the pancreas: imaging findings with pathologic correlation. AJR Am J Roentgenol. 2009;193(1):136–42.

Crippa S, Salvia R, Warshaw AL, Domínguez I, Bassi C, Falconi M, et al. Mucinous cystic neoplasm of the pancreas is not an aggressive entity: lessons from 163 resected patients. Ann Surg. 2008;247(4):571–9.

Gupta R, Mortelé KJ, Tatli S, Girshman J, Glickman JN, Levy AD, et al. Pancreatic intraductal papillary mucinous neoplasms: role of CT in predicting pathologic subtypes. AJR Am J Roentgenol. 2008;191(5):1458–64.

Irie H, Honda H, Aibe H, Kuroiwa T, Yoshimitsu K, Shinozaki K, et al. MR cholangiopancreatographic differentiation of benign and malignant intraductal mucin-producing tumors of the pancreas. AJR Am J Roentgenol. 2000;174(5):1403–8.

Irie H, Yoshimitsu K, Aibe H, Tajima T, Nishie A, Nakayama T, et al. Natural history of pancreatic intraductal papillary mucinous tumor of branch duct type: follow-up study by magnetic resonance cholangiopancreatography. J Comput Assist Tomogr. 2004;28(1):117–22.

Ishigami K, Yoshimitsu K, Irie H, Shinozaki K, Nagata S, Yamaguchi K, et al. Imaging of intraductal tubular tumors of the pancreas. AJR Am J Roentgenol. 2008;191(6):1836–40.

Ishigami K, Yoshimitsu K, Irie H, Tajima T, Asayama Y, Nishie A, et al. Diagnostic value of the delayed phase image for iso-attenuating pancreatic carcinomas in the pancreatic parenchymal phase on multidetector computed tomography. Eur J Radiol. 2009;69(1):139–46.

Kawamoto S, Lawler LP, Horton KM, Eng J, Hruban RH, Fishman EK. MDCT of intraductal papillary mucinous neoplasm of the pancreas: evaluation of features predictive of invasive carcinoma. AJR Am J Roentgenol. 2006;186(3):687–95.

Kimura W, Moriya T, Hanada K, Abe H, Yanagisawa A, Fukushima N, et al. Multicenter study of serous cystic neoplasm of the Japan pancreas society. Pancreas. 2012;41(3):380–7.

Laffan TA, Horton KM, Klein AP, Berlanstein B, Siegelman SS, Kawamoto S, et al. Prevalence of unsuspected pancreatic cysts on MDCT. AJR Am J Roentgenol. 2008;191(3):802–7.

Manfredi R, Graziani R, Motton M, Mantovani W, Baltieri S, Tognolini A, et al. Main pancreatic duct intraductal papillary mucinous neoplasms: accuracy of MR imaging in differentiation between benign and malignant tumors compared with histopathologic analysis. Radiology. 2009;253(1):106–15.

McNulty NJ, Francis IR, Platt JF, Cohan RH, Korobkin M, Gebremariam A. Multi–detector row helical CT of the pancreas: effect of contrast-enhanced multiphasic imaging on enhancement of the pancreas, peripancreatic vasculature, and pancreatic adenocarcinoma. Radiology. 2001;220(1):97–102.

Mori Y, Ohtsuka T, Kono H, Ideno N, Aso T, Nagayoshi Y, et al. Management strategy for multifocal branch duct intraductal papillary mucinous neoplasms of the pancreas. Pancreas. 2012;41(7):1008–12.

Nara S, Onaya H, Hiraoka N, Shimada K, Sano T, Sakamoto Y, et al. Preoperative evaluation of invasive and noninvasive intraductal papillary-mucinous neoplasms of the pancreas: clinical, radiological, and pathological analysis of 123 cases. Pancreas. 2009;38(1):8–16.

Ogawa H, Itoh S, Ikeda M, Suzuki K, Naganawa S. Intraductal papillary mucinous neoplasm of the pancreas: assessment of the likelihood of invasiveness with multisection CT. Radiology. 2008;248(3):876–86.

Pedrosa I, Boparai D. Imaging considerations in intraductal papillary mucinous neoplasms of the pancreas. World J Gastrointest Surg. 2010;2(10):324–30.

Reddy RP, Smyrk TC, Zapiach M, Levy MJ, Pearson RK, Clain JE, et al. Pancreatic mucinous cystic neoplasm defined by ovarian stroma: demographics, clinical features, and prevalence of cancer. Clin Gastroenterol Hepatol. 2004;2(11):1026–31.

Spinelli KS, Fromwiller TE, Daniel RA, Kiely JM, Nakeeb A, Komorowski RA, et al. Cystic pancreatic neoplasms: observe or operate. Ann Surg. 2004;239(5):651–7. discussion 657–9.

Sugiyama M, Izumisato Y, Abe N, Masaki T, Mori T, Atomi Y. Predictive factors for malignancy in intraductal papillary-mucinous tumours of the pancreas. Br J Surg. 2003;90(10):1244–9.

Tanaka M, Fernández-del Castillo C, Adsay V, Chari S, Falconi M, Jang JY, et al. International association of pancreatology. International consensus guidelines 2012 for the management of IPMN and MCN of the pancreas. Pancreatology. 2012;12(3):183–97.

Vullierme MP, Giraud-Cohen M, Hammel P, Sauvanet A, Couvelard A, O'Toole D, et al. Malignant intraductal papillary mucinous neoplasm of the pancreas: in situ versus invasive carcinoma surgical resectability. Radiology. 2007;245(2):483–90.

Waters JA, Schmidt CM, Pinchot JW, White PB, Cummings OW, Pitt HA, et al. CT vs MRCP: optimal classification of IPMN type and extent. J Gastrointest Surg. 2008;12(1):101–9.

Yamaguchi K, Ogawa Y, Chijiiwa K, Tanaka M. Mucin-hypersecreting tumors of the pancreas: assessing the grade of malignancy preoperatively. Am J Surg. 1996;171(4):427–31.

Yamaguchi H, Ishigami K, Inoue T, Eguchi T, Nagata S, Kuroda Y, et al. Three cases of serous oligocystic adenomas of the pancreas; evaluation of cyst wall thickness for preoperative differentiation from mucinous cystic neoplasms. J Gastrointest Cancer. 2007;38(1):52–8.

Yamaguchi H, Shimizu M, Ban S, Koyama I, Hatori T, Fujita I, et al. Intraductal tubulopapillary neoplasms of the pancreas distinct from pancreatic intraepithelial neoplasia and intraductal papillary mucinous neoplasms. Am J Surg Pathol. 2009;33(8):1164–72.

Yamaguchi K, Kanemitsu S, Hatori T, Maguchi H, Shimizu Y, Tada M, et al. Pancreatic ductal adenocarcinoma derived from IPMN and pancreatic ductal adenocarcinoma concomitant with IPMN. Pancreas. 2011;40(4):571–80.

Yamao K, Yanagisawa A, Takahashi K, Kimura W, Doi R, Fukushima N, et al. Clinicopathological features and prognosis of mucinous cystic neoplasm with ovarian-type stroma: a multi-institutional study of the Japan pancreas society. Pancreas. 2011;40(1):67–71.

Yoon LS, Catalano OA, Fritz S, Ferrone CR, Hahn PF, Sahani DV. Another dimension in magnetic resonance cholangiopancreatography: comparison of 2- and 3-dimensional magnetic resonance cholangiopancreatography for the evaluation of intraductal papillary mucinous neoplasm of the pancreas. J Comput Assist Tomogr. 2009;33(3):363–8.

Yoon SH, Lee JM, Cho JY, Lee KB, Kim JE, Moon SK, et al. Small (≤20 mm) pancreatic adenocarcinomas: analysis of enhancement patterns and secondary signs with multiphasic multidetector CT. Radiology. 2011;259(2):442–52.

Zhang XM, Mitchell DG, Dohke M, Holland GA, Parker L. Pancreatic cysts: depiction on single-shot fast spin-echo MR images. Radiology. 2002;223(2):547–53.

Chapter 6
Endosonography

Susumu Hijioka, Vikram Bhatia, and Kenji Yamao

Abstract Endoscopic ultrasound (EUS) is an important modality for the evaluation of patients with a suspicion of intraductal papillary mucinous neoplasms (IPMNs) of the pancreas. EUS imaging from the stomach and duodenum can demonstrate the entire pancreatic gland with a high spatial resolution. It can distinguish IPMN from other cystic lesions, detect malignant degeneration in IPMN (IPMC), and is invaluable to follow up these patients. From a clinical viewpoint, the key issue is whether an individual patient with IPMN should undergo surgery or can be managed conservatively. EUS helps in this decision by demonstrating the presence or absence of "high-risk stigmata of malignancy" or "worrisome features," as per the revised IPMN/MCN Consensus Guidelines 2012. It is important to detect mural nodules (MNs), which correspond to macroscopic papillary growth pattern of these tumors, and measure their precise diameter as an indicator of the malignant potential of BD- or mixed-type IPMN. EUS can depict MNs as slightly hyperechoic papillary projections. The differentiation between MNs and mucin plugs can be challenging, and contrast-enhanced EUS imaging may be needed to demonstrate enhancement of the former.

There are two echo patterns of pancreatic ductal adenocarcinoma (PDAC) derived from IPMN on EUS: mixed-echo pattern which is a feature of mucinous carcinoma usually derived from intestinal type and solid-echo pattern which is a feature of tubular adenocarcinoma usually derived from gastric type of IPMN. The latter is similar to the common PDAC. Since recent studies have shown that patients with IPMN have high risk for development of PDAC, it is vital to carefully evaluate the entire pancreas during follow-up.

S. Hijioka • K. Yamao (✉)
Department of Gastroenterology, Aichi Cancer Center Hospital,
1-1 Kanokoden, Chikusa-ku, Nagoya City, Aichi 464-8681, Japan
e-mail: kyamao@aichi-cc.jp

V. Bhatia
Department of Medical Hepatology, Institute of Liver and Biliary Sciences, Delhi, India

M. Tanaka (ed.), *Intraductal Papillary Mucinous Neoplasm of the Pancreas*,
DOI 10.1007/978-4-431-54472-2_6, © Springer Japan 2014

Keywords Endoscopic ultrasonography (EUS) • Intraductal papillary mucinous carcinoma (IPMC) • Intraductal papillary mucinous neoplasm (IPMN) • IPMN/MCN consensus guidelines • Pancreatic ductal adenocarcinoma (PDAC)

6.1 Introduction

Endoscopic ultrasonography (EUS) includes probes with two methods of imaging: radial instruments with 360° imaging perpendicular to the long axis; and convex instruments with imaging plane parallel to the long axis of the instrument. The former only allows diagnostic imaging, whereas the latter was developed for fine-needle aspiration (FNA) (Inui et al. 2004; Yamao et al. 2007). EUS operates at a high ultrasound frequencies, with imaging from the stomach or duodenum, providing high-resolution, real-time imaging of the pancreas. This modality therefore plays an important role in the evaluation of pancreatic diseases.

In this chapter, we describe the diagnosis of intraductal papillary mucinous neoplasm (IPMN) using EUS with a special emphasis on (1) differentiation from other cystic lesions, (2) detailed morphologic description of IPMN, and (3) EUS-based follow-up protocol.

6.2 Differential Diagnosis of IPMN from Other Cystic Lesions

With advances in cross-sectional imaging techniques, IPMN and other pancreatic cysts are frequently detected by ultrasound (US), computed tomographic (CT) scanning, or magnetic resonance imaging (MRI). Although these imaging modalities are very sensitive for the detection of pancreatic cystic lesions, they are suboptimal for characterization of the cyst type. EUS remains an essential modality for differentiation of IPMN from other cystic lesions. There are many reports on EUS findings in cystic lesions of the pancreas (Sedlack et al. 2002; Song et al. 2003; Brugge 2000; Ahmad et al. 2003; Kim et al. 2010; Okabe et al. 2011; Sahani et al. 2013). Diagnosis based on EUS features requires close attention to the size and number of cysts, contour of the cystic lesion, morphology of the cyst wall, internal contents of the cysts, presence or absence of communication between the cyst and the pancreatic duct, as well as the coexistence of any other pancreatic pathology.

When the main pancreatic duct (MPD) is dilated along with the presence of multilocular cysts with typical "bunch of grapes" appearance, the diagnosis of IPMN is relatively easy. However, when mucinous secretions and hence ductal dilatation are minimal, IPMN can be difficult to differentiate from other cystic conditions, such as macrocystic serous cystic neoplasm (SCN) and retention cysts. In this situation, EUS depiction of communication between a cyst and the MPD is indicative of IPMN. Also use of sonographic contrast agents like Sonazoid® can help to distinguish debris in a retention cyst from mural nodules (MNs) in an IPMN cyst (Fig. 6.1).

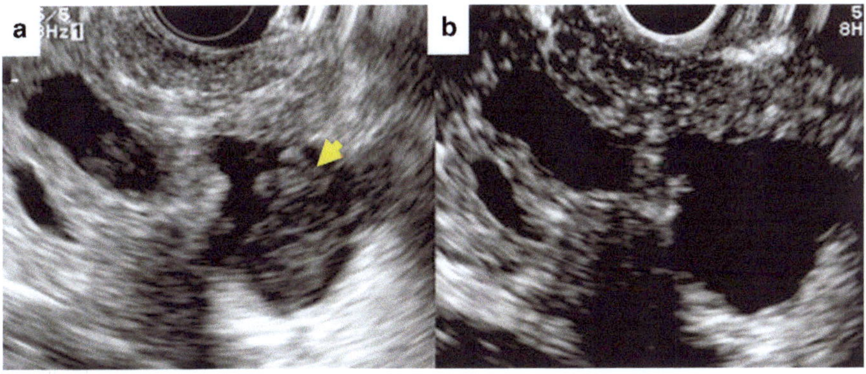

Fig. 6.1 Pseudocyst with debris. The use of contrast agents revealed the absence of blood flow signals in the cyst, that excludes mural nodules and we can diagnose debris (*arrow*)

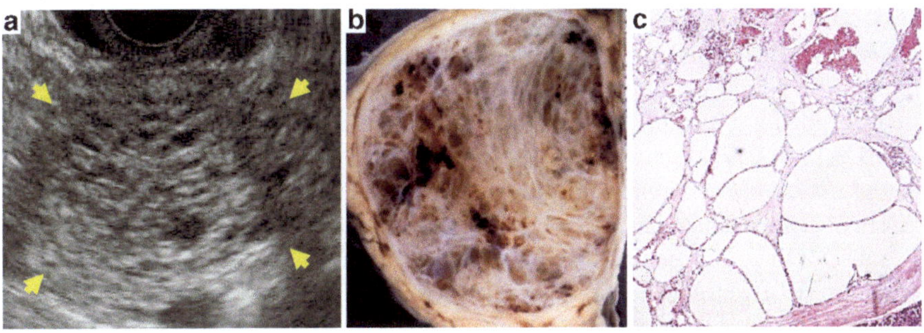

Fig. 6.2 Serous cystic neoplasm (SCN) microcystic type. EUS (*arrow*) shows honeycomb-like pattern as a result of accumulation of microcysts

The typical microcystic SCNs have a honeycomb-like aggregation of tiny cysts, and this appearance on EUS is a characteristic (Fig. 6.2). Differentiating branch duct IPMN (BD-IPMN) from mucinous cystic neoplasms (MCN) can be sometimes problematic. MCN are typically round to ovoid tumor, having a typical cyst-in-cyst pattern, with a common external thick wall (Fig. 6.3). Differentiating MCN from IPMN therefore relies on whether the cyst structure is directed inwards or outwards. Retention cysts and pseudocysts are formed when pancreatic duct is obstructed by a solid tumor such as PDAC. These cysts can be misdiagnosed as IPMNs, particularly when the obstructing solid component is small. Thus, meticulous EUS observation is essential to look for any solid lesion near the cysts.

Ahmad et al. (2003) reported that the EUS diagnosis was correct in 40–93 % cases, among eight endoscopists, depending on their experience in terms of number of cases that they had performed and also on their technical skills. Thus EUS is an operator-dependent examination, and there may be considerable variability in the ability to correctly differentiate between benign and malignant lesions (Sedlack et al. 2002; Hernandez et al. 2002; Canto et al. 2004; Brugge et al. 2004; Ahmad et al. 2003; Khalid and Brugge 2007).

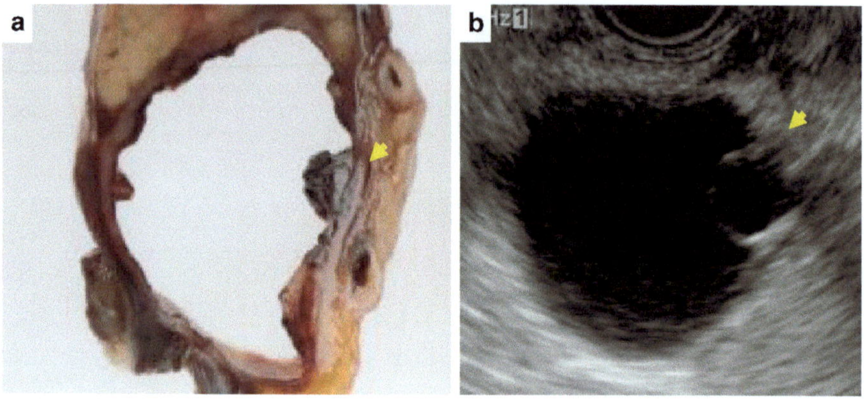

Fig. 6.3 Mucinous cystic neoplasms (MCN) has a typical cyst-in-cyst pattern with a common external thick wall

For the differential diagnosis of pancreatic cystic lesions and the grading of tumors, cyst fluid cytology, and measurements of pancreatic enzymes (amylase, lipase) and tumor markers like carcinoembryonic antigen (CEA), carbohydrate antigen (CA19-9, CA125, etc.) in the cyst fluid is widely used (Brugge et al. 2004). One of the noticeable differences in the diagnostic approach to pancreatic cystic neoplasms between Japan and other countries is the use of pancreatic cyst aspiration. Because of the presence of a case report of post-EUS-FNA tumor seeding (Hirooka et al. 2003), current Japanese consensus is that aspiration of pancreatic cystic lesions should be avoided when an MCN is suspected (Yamao et al. 2009).

6.3 Detailed Morphological Examination of IPMN

6.3.1 Imaging BD-Type and Mixed-Type IPMN (Figs. 6.4 and 6.5)

One of the key features of IPMN is dilatation of a branch duct (BD) or main duct (MD) due to proliferative papillary tumors themselves or large amounts of secreted intraductal mucin. Accordingly, the size of IPMN depends on the diameter of the dilated BD, MD, and MNs. An accurate measurement of the dilated BD and the MD diameters is important for defining BD- and mixed-type IPMN. The diameter of dilated ducts can be measured by either MDCT or MRCP, but only EUS is sufficiently accurate for measuring the size of MNs. Presence of MNs is considered to be the most reliable indicator of whether an IPMN tumor is benign or malignant, and this issue has been the subject of numerous studies. However, a cutoff diameter for differentiating benign from malignant nodules has been controversial and ranges between 3 and 10 mm.

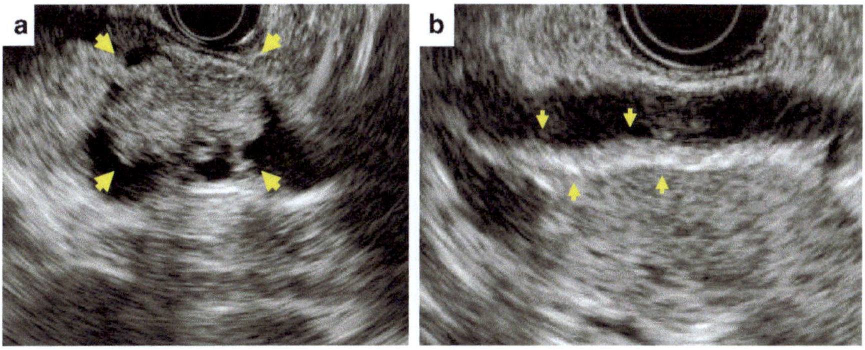

Fig. 6.4 EUS findings of "worrisome features" with the high malignancy potential. (**a**) obvious mural nodules (*arrow*), (**b**) lesions in the main duct (*arrow*)

The revised international guidelines 2012 (Tanaka et al. 2012) recommend that cysts with worrisome features should undergo a detailed evaluation by EUS. Surgery is indicated if EUS reveals obvious MNs (Fig. 6.4a), or main duct lesions (Fig. 6.4b), and when cyst fluid cytology reveals malignancy. These guidelines define high-risk stigmata in BD- and mixed-type IPMN as the presence of obstructive jaundice, an enhancing solid component (Fig. 6.5e), and a main duct diameter ≥10 mm. A notable change from the previous guidelines is that side-branch dilatation of ≥3 cm in BD-IPMN, which was an indication for surgery earlier (Tanaka et al. 2006), is now considered a worrisome feature. These lesions should be carefully assessed for the presence of MNs by EUS. In all of these situations, EUS is a key modality for risk stratification and classification of IPMN lesions.

MNs appear as hyperechoic wall-based structures on EUS, because the papillary structures comprising the MN scatter the ultrasound waves (Fig. 6.6). It is important to distinguish MNs from protein plaques, viscous mucin, or debris. Protein plaques can be differentiated by their characteristic annular hyperechoic appearance with a low echoic central part (Fig. 6.7), whereas discriminating mucin from MNs is difficult by B-mode imaging. Caution is needed in this regard, because misdiagnosis of mucin as a nodule will lead to an overdiagnosis of malignancy. The use of ultrasound contrast agents, such as Sonazoid®, can rule out MNs by the absence of blood flow signals in the intra-cystic structure (Fig. 6.8), thus increasing the diagnostic precision of EUS (Ohno et al. 2009).

6.3.2 Imaging of MD-Type IPMN

Main duct IPMN (MD-IPMN) is defined by segmental or diffuse MD dilatation to ≥6 mm, without branch duct dilatation >5 mm (Tanaka et al. 2006). Furthermore, an MD diameter ≥10 mm is considered as high-risk stigmata, as per the international consensus guidelines (Tanaka et al. 2012), and resection is recommended in

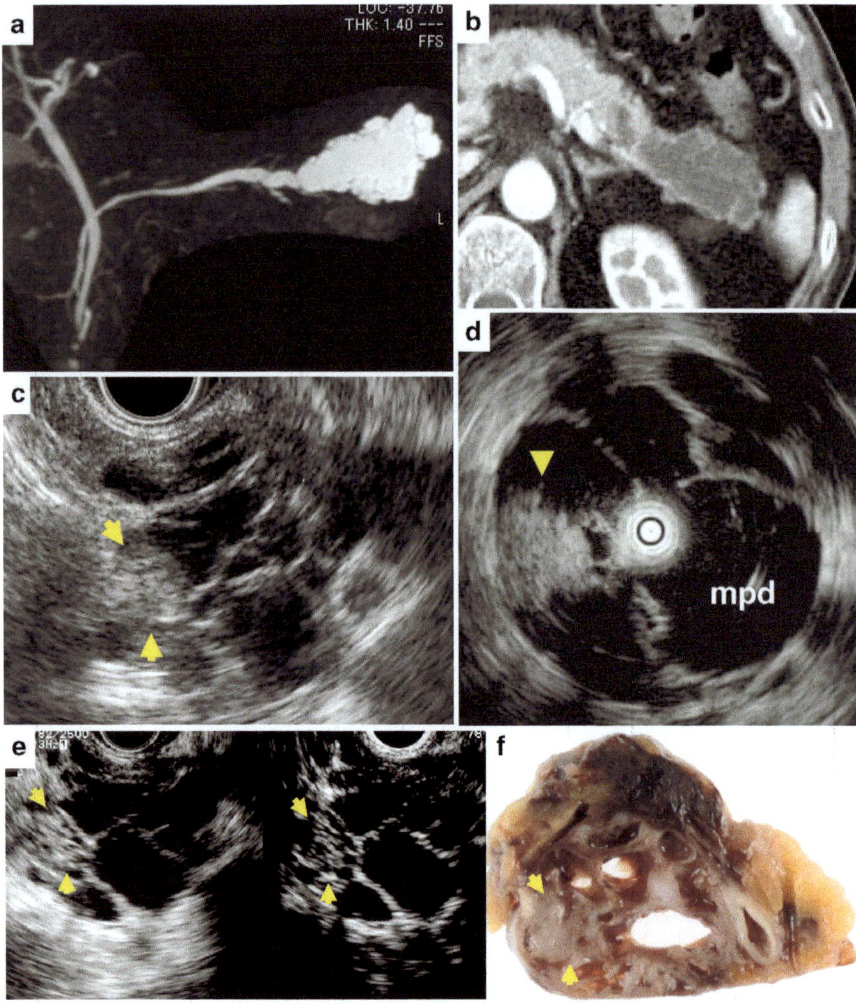

Fig. 6.5 Mixed-type IPMN (MPD10 mm with dilated branch) in the tail. EUS and IDUS shows hyperechoic mass (*arrow*) in the dilated branch, The use of contrast agents revealed blood flow signals in the mass, it allows to diagnose mural nodules

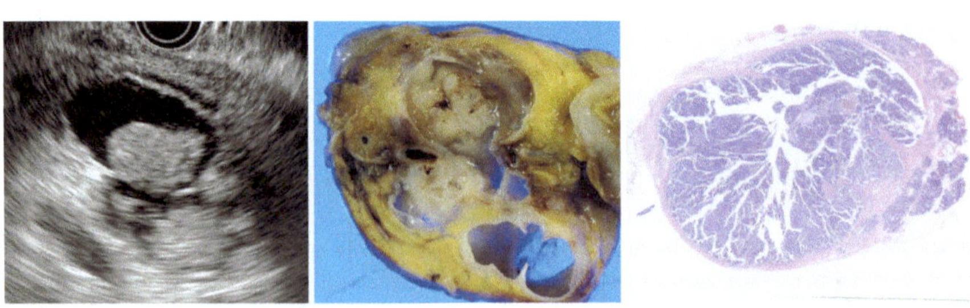

Fig. 6.6 MNs in the dilated branch (mixed-typeIPMN). EUS detects the MNs as hyperechoic masses because of ultrasonic scattering by the papillary structures

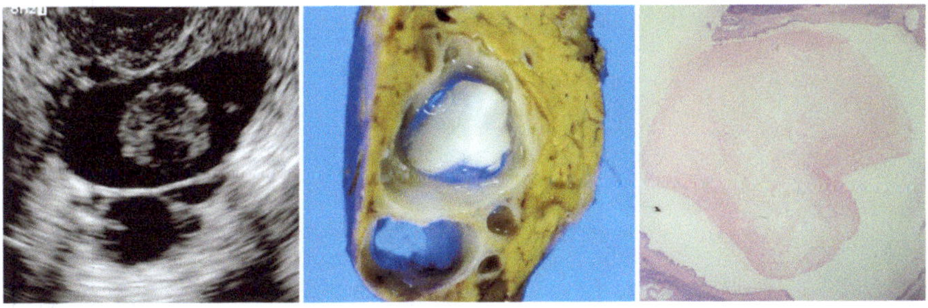

Fig. 6.7 Protein plaque in the dilated branch (BD-PMN). EUS finds protein plaque as annular hyperechoic lesion with low echoic central part

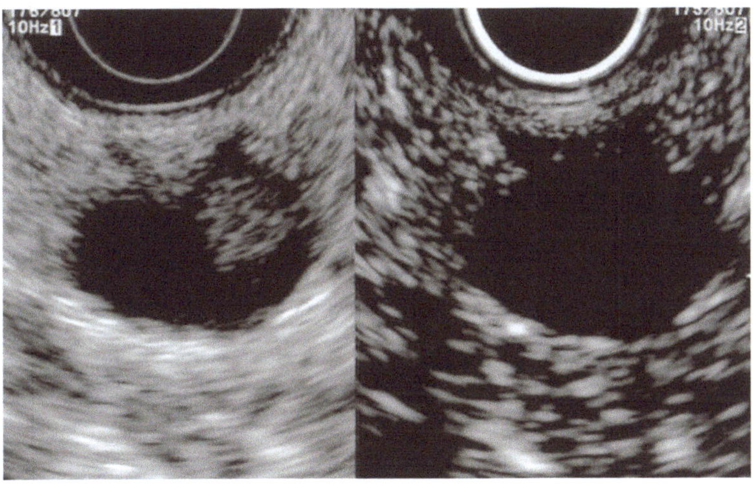

Fig. 6.8 Debris the use of contrast agents revealed the absence of blood flow signals in the cyst, it allows to exclude mural nodules and to diagnose debris (*arrow*)

such cases. It is important to observe the entire pancreatic duct till the ampulla of Vater, to rule out upstream ductal dilatation due to chronic pancreatitis or obstruction by a PDAC.

Large papillary projections in a dilated MD can be evaluated using CT or MRCP, but EUS may be the most suitable investigation for smaller nodules (Fig. 6.9). MD-IPMN has a tendency for superficial intraductal extension. Hence, an accurate preoperative assessment of the longitudinal extent of the disease is important to decide the magnitude of pancreatic resection, such as total pancreatectomy or partial pancreatectomy. Intraductal ultrasound (IDUS) and peroral pancreatoscopy (POPS) are other useful modalities for determining the extent of intraductal superficial lesions (Fig. 6.10).

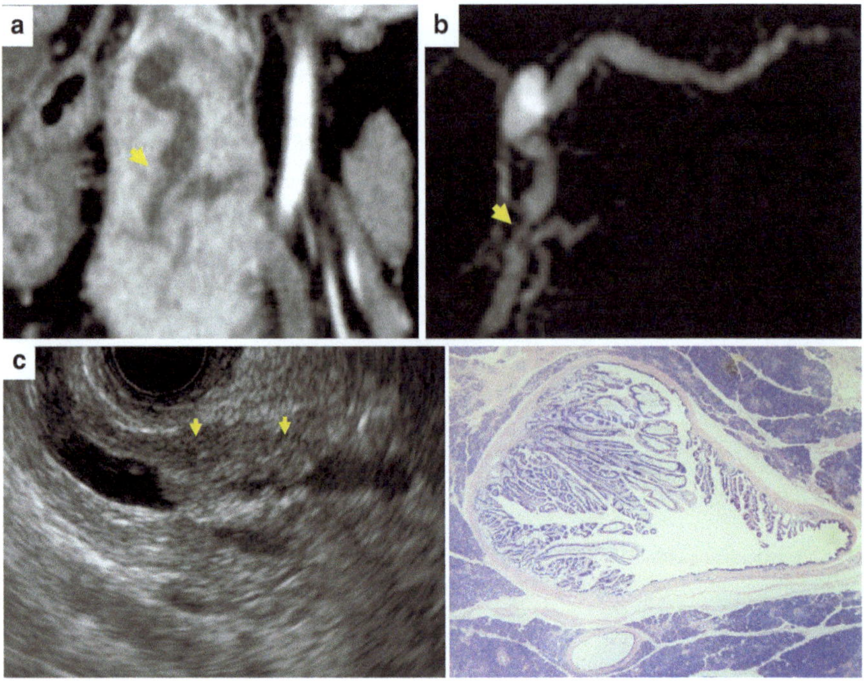

Fig. 6.9 MD-IPMN CT and MRCP found dilatation of MPD and stenosis in pancreatic head but could not detect the mural nodule. EUS could detect the MN in MPD

6.3.3 Imaging of PDAC Derived from IPMN

The Japan Pancreas Society (JPS) formed a committee to resolve the clinical and pathological issues associated with PDAC derived from IPMN and PDAC concomitant with IPMN. This committee proposed new definitions of three categories based on the topological relationship of two conditions and presence or absence of a histological transition between these conditions (Yamaguchi et al. 2011):

(a) PDAC derived from IPMN (PDAC is clearly derived from IPMN.)
(b) PDAC concomitant with IPMN (PDAC is obviously different from the IPMN lesions.)
(c) PDAC of undetermined relationship with IPMN (whether PDAC was derived from IPMN or whether PDAC was concomitant with IPMN could not be determined, because there was no histological transition between the two diseases).

With regard to the histological subtypes, approximately one-third of PDAC derived from IPMN (41/122) were mucinous carcinomas, while most of PDAC concomitant with IPMN (28/31) were tubular adenocarcinomas, similar to the usual PDAC. Accordingly mucinous carcinoma was more frequently seen as the histological subtype when the PDAC was derived from IPMN, than when PDAC occurred

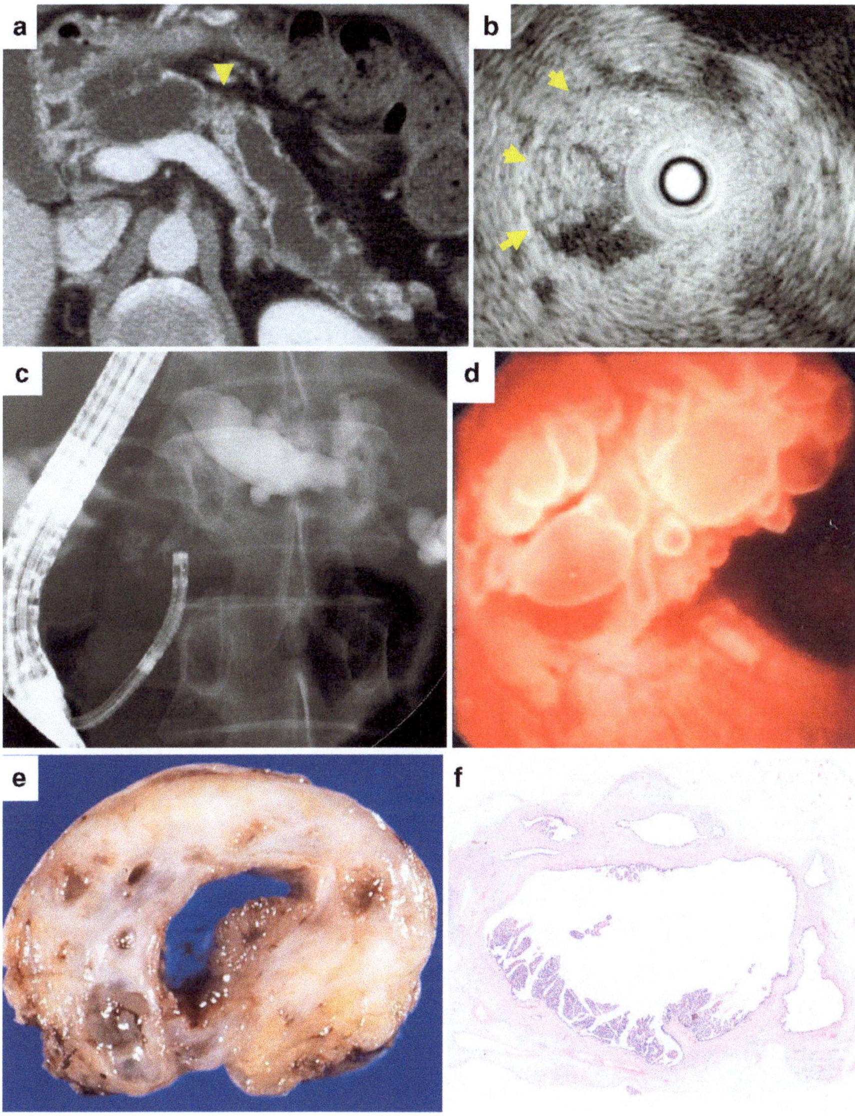

Fig. 6.10 (**a**) MD-IPMN type (**b**) IDUS, (**c**, **d**) POCS, (**e**, **f**) papirally tumor with adenoma in MPD

either alone or concomitantly with IPMN (Yamaguchi et al. 2011). During EUS evaluation of PDAC derived from IPMN, two echo patterns can be observed: Mucinous carcinoma derived from intestinal type usually shows a mixed-echo pattern (Fig. 6.11). On the other hand, tubular adenocarcinoma, which is similar to common PDAC and is usually derived from gastric type, shows a solid-echo pattern (Kobayashi et al. 2005) (Fig. 6.12).

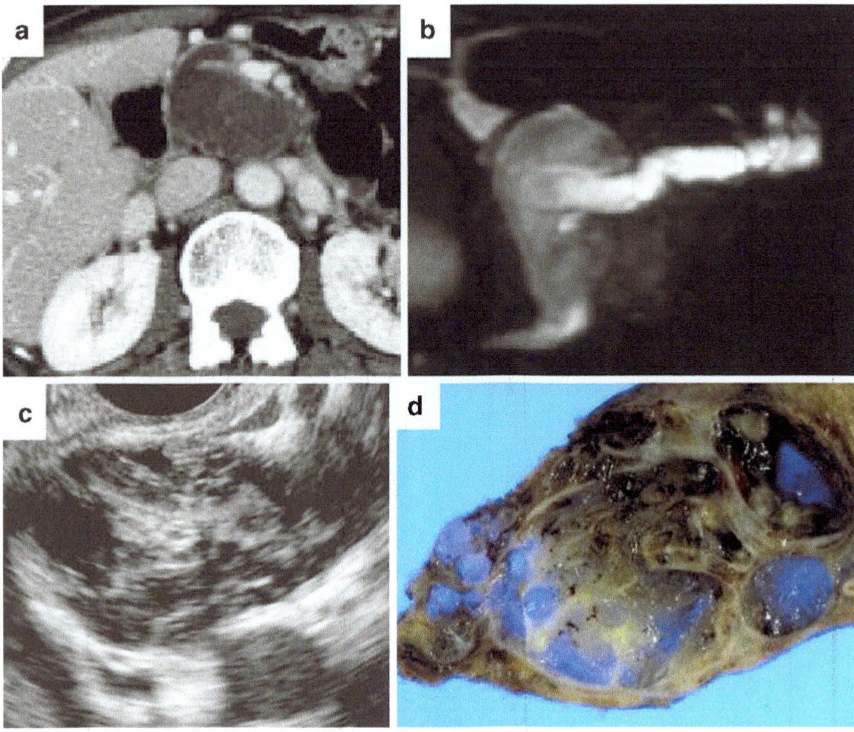

Fig. 6.11 Mucinous carcinoma derived from IPMN. EUS shows mixed-echo pattern

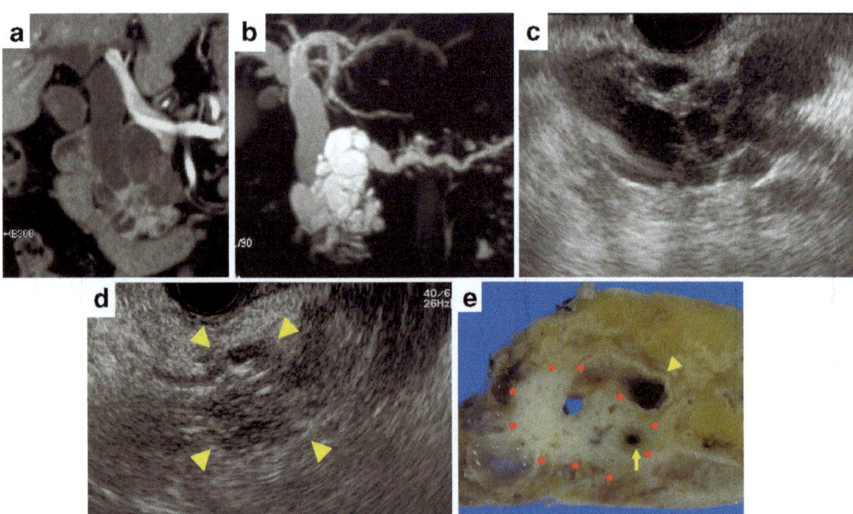

Fig. 6.12 Tubular adenocarcinoma derived from IPMN. EUS shows solid-echo pattern similar to common PDAC

6.4 Protocol for Follow-Up of Patients with IPMN

When both high-risk stigmata and worrisome features are absent, no MNs are detected by EUS examination, lesions localized in the BD, and pancreatic juice cytology findings are negative, the revised international guidelines specify the follow-up protocol depending on the cyst size (1–2 cm or 2–3 cm). The recommended imaging modalities for follow-up of these patients are CT/MRI and EUS (Tanaka et al. 2012).

A large natural history study of BD-IPMN from Japan (Maguchi et al. 2011), based on a nationwide survey, found that disease progression rate was 18 %, whereas stable disease was seen in 82 % of 349 patients without MNs at the initial diagnosis, over a mean observation period of 3.7 years. The rate of IPMC occurring in these patients was 2.5 % (Fig. 6.13).

Recently high rates of PDAC concomitant with IPMN have been reported (2.0–9.3 %). Hence, patients with IPMN should be regarded as a high-risk group for developing PDAC (Fig. 6.14).

These observations highlight the importance of not only evaluating the IPMN lesions but also carefully observing the entire pancreas during the follow-up EUS studies, so as not to miss PDAC. Regular EUS evaluations can allow early detection of PDAC in such cases.

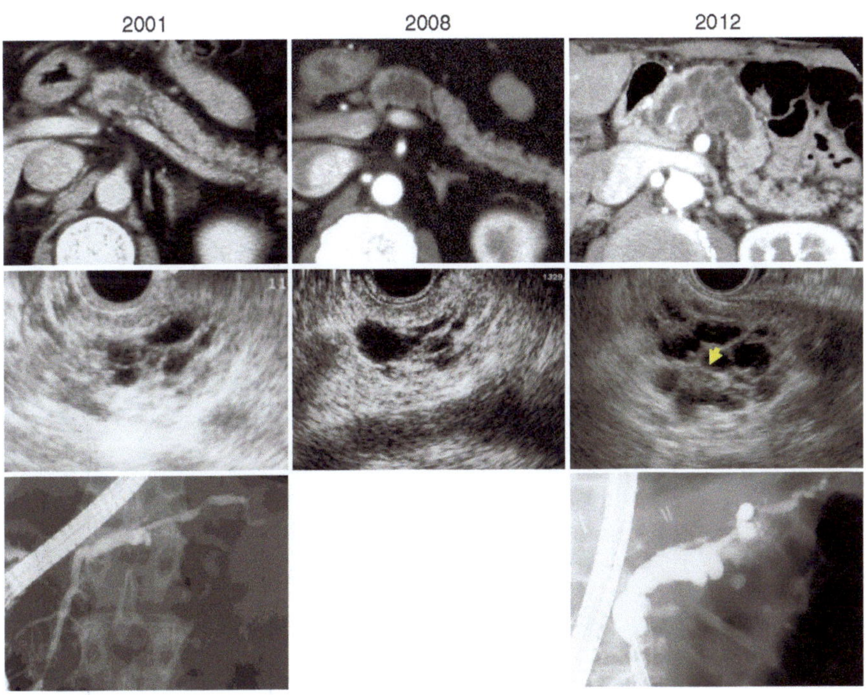

Fig. 6.13 IPMC (carcinoma in situ) after following up for 10 years, 2001: cyst size 15 mm MPD 6 mm 2008: cyst size 25 mm, 2012: cyst size 40 mm with thickened wall, MPD 10 mm

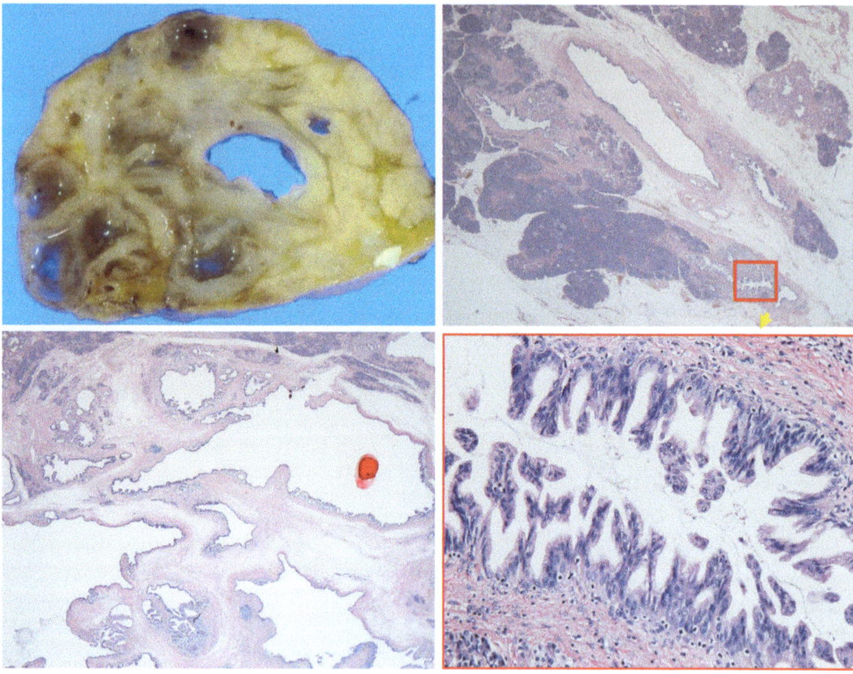

Fig. 6.13 (continued)

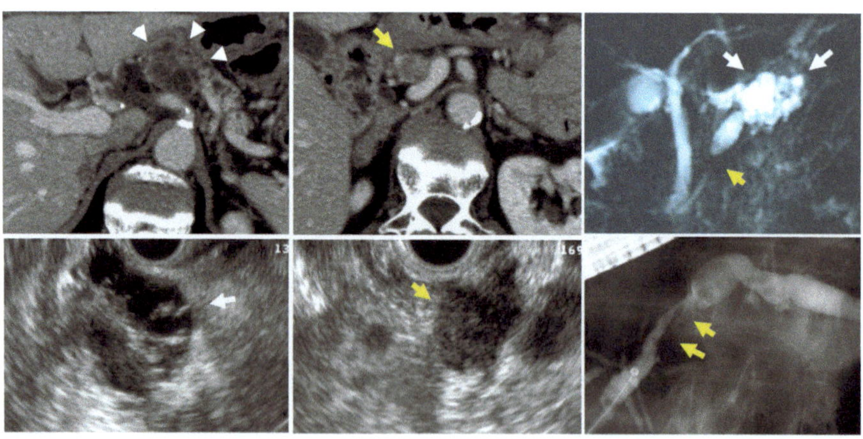

Fig. 6.14 PDAC concomitant with IPMN. This case has been followed up during 5 years because of BD-IPMN. 12 mm mass in the pancreas head was appeared after 5 years have passed. Pancreatectomy revealed T1 pancreas cancer

References

Ahmad NA, Kochman ML, Brensinger C, et al. Interobserver agreement among endosonographers for the diagnosis of neoplastic versus non-neoplastic pancreatic cystic lesions. Gastrointest Endosc. 2003;58:59–64.

Brugge WR. The role of EUS in the diagnosis of cystic lesions of the pancreas. Gastrointest Endosc. 2000;52:18.

Brugge WR, Lewandrowski K, Lee-Lewandrowski E, et al. Diagnosis of pancreatic cystic neoplasms: a report of the cooperative pancreatic cyst study. Gastroenterology. 2004;126:1330–6.

Canto MI, Goggins M, Yeo CJ, et al. Screening for pancreatic neoplasia in high-risk individuals: an EUS-based approach. Clin Gastroenterol Hepatol. 2004;2:606–21.

Hernandez LV, Mishra G, Forsmark C, et al. Role of endoscopic ultrasound (EUS) and EUS-guided fine needle aspiration in the diagnosis and treatment of cystic lesions of the pancreas. Pancreas. 2002;25:222–8.

Hirooka Y, Goto H, Itoh A, et al. Case of intraductal papillary mucinous tumor in which endosonography-guided fine-needle aspiration biopsy caused dissemination. J Gastroenterol Hepatol. 2003;18:1323–4.

Inui K, Kida M, Fujita N, et al. Standard imaging techniques in the pancreatobiliary region using radial scanning endoscopic ultrasonography. Dig Endosc. 2004;16:S118–33.

Khalid A, Brugge W. ACG practice guidelines for the diagnosis and management of neoplastic pancreatic cysts. Am J Gastroenterol. 2007;102:2339–49.

Kim YC, Choi JY, Chung YE, et al. Comparison of MRI and endoscopic ultrasound in the characterization of pancreatic cystic lesions. AJR Am J Roentgenol. 2010;195:947–52.

Kobayashi G, Fujita N, Noda Y, et al. Mode of progression of intraductal papillary-mucinous tumor of the pancreas: analysis of patients with follow-up by EUS. J Gastroenterol. 2005;40:744–51.

Maguchi H, Tanno S, Mizuno N, et al. Natural history of branch duct intraductal papillary mucinous neoplasms of the pancreas: a multicenter study in Japan. Pancreas. 2011;40:364.

Ohno E, Hirooka Y, Itoh A, et al. Intraductal papillary mucinous neoplasms of the pancreas: differentiation of malignant and benign tumors by endoscopic ultrasound findings of mural nodules. Ann Surg. 2009;249:628–34.

Okabe Y, Kaji R, Ishida Y, et al. The management of the pancreatic cystic neoplasm: the role of the EUS in Japan. Dig Endosc. 2011;23:39–42.

Sahani DV, Kambadakone A, Macari M, et al. Diagnosis and management of cystic pancreatic lesions. AJR Am J Roentgenol. 2013;200:343–54.

Sedlack R, Affi A, Vazquez-Sequeiros E, et al. Utility of EUS in the evaluation of cystic pancreatic lesions. Gastrointest Endosc. 2002;56:543–7.

Song MH, Lee SK, Kim MH, et al. EUS in the evaluation of pancreatic cystic lesions. Gastrointest Endosc. 2003;57:891–6.

Tanaka M, Chari S, Adsay V, et al. International consensus guidelines for management of intraductal papillary mucinous neoplasms and mucinous cystic neoplasms of the pancreas. Pancreatology. 2006;6:17–32.

Tanaka M, Castillo CF, Adsay V, et al. International consensus guidelines 2012 for the management of IPMN and MCN of the pancreas. Pancreatology. 2012;12:183–97.

Yamaguchi K, Kanemitsu S, Hatori T, et al. Pancreatic ductal adenocarcinoma derived from IPMN and pancreatic ductal adenocarcinoma concomitant with IPMN. Pancreas. 2011;40:571–80.

Yamao K, Irisawa A, Inoue H, et al. Standard imaging techniques of endoscopic ultrasound-guided fine-needle aspiration using a curved linear array echoendoscope. Dig Endosc. 2007;19:S180–205.

Yamao K, Mizuno N, Takagi T, et al. How I do it and when I use (and do not use) EUS-FNA. Gastrointest Endosc. 2009;69.

Chapter 7
Diagnostic Investigation of Pancreatic Cyst Fluid

Martha Bishop Pitman

Abstract Determining whether a pancreatic cyst is mucinous or non-mucinous and then benign or malignant are the key clinical questions that drive patient management. The analysis of pancreatic cyst fluid is a vital component of the multimodal approach to preoperative evaluation that answers these questions. Methods of evaluating cyst fluid include biochemical, molecular, and cytological analysis, which, in combination, can accurately identify cyst type and grade in most instances. Preoperative diagnosis of a high-grade IPMN (high-grade dysplasia or adenocarcinoma (invasive carcinoma)) will result in resection, whereas a low-grade IPMN by imaging and cyst fluid analysis may be followed conservatively. This chapter addresses how to handle aspirated cyst fluid for cytological and ancillary testing and the clinical utility of each test.

Keywords Cyst fluid analysis • Cytology • Endoscopic ultrasound-guided fine-needle aspiration • EUS-FNA • IPMN • Pancreas

7.1 Introduction and Background

Preoperative fine-needle aspiration (FNA) of pancreatic cysts with cyst fluid analysis (CFA) is performed to assess the nature of the pancreatic cyst, not only for the distinction between a non-mucinous and mucinous cyst but also for the assessment of malignancy. The goal of preoperative evaluation is to determine patient management, and the answer to these key clinical questions—cyst type and grade—will directly impact the need for surgical intervention. FNA is most often performed with endoscopic ultrasound (EUS) guidance as EUS allows for a high-resolution

M.B. Pitman (✉)
Massachusetts General Hospital, Boston, MA 02114, USA

Harvard Medical School, Boston, MA 02115, USA
e-mail: mpitman@partners.org

M. Tanaka (ed.), *Intraductal Papillary Mucinous Neoplasm of the Pancreas*,
DOI 10.1007/978-4-431-54472-2_7,

evaluation of the cyst while at the same time providing a means to aspirate the cyst contents for biochemical, molecular, and cytological analysis. CFA provides a glimpse into the cyst that is not attainable any other way including with high-resolution imaging. When conservative management is the goal due to a clinical diagnosis of a non-mucinous or low-risk mucinous cyst from imaging studies, then CFA becomes even more critical as a component of a triple negative test (Wu et al. 2012).

Early studies of CFA from the 1980s evaluated many different cyst fluid characteristics, including viscosity and biochemical and tumor markers such as CA19-9, CA 72-4 (TAG-72), CA15-3, carcinoembryonic antigen (CEA), CA 125, and amylase (Tatsuta et al. 1986; Lewandrowski et al. 1992; Alles et al. 1994; Rubin et al. 1994; Hammel et al. 1995; Lewandrowski et al. 1995). Today viscosity is still important by gross inspection, but, according to a recent study from a single institution, CEA is the most accurate marker of a mucinous cyst and cytology is the most accurate marker for malignancy (Cizginer et al. 2011). Molecular markers such as *KRAS* and *GNAS* support the classification of the cyst as mucinous and are useful when CEA is not elevated or on the rare occasion when an elevated CEA is associated with a non-mucinous cyst, and to distinguish MCN from IPMN. However, molecular markers do not distinguish benign from malignant cysts (Khalid et al. 2009; Wu et al. 2011).

7.1.1 EUS-FNA Technique

EUS-FNA is a low-risk procedure that produces high-resolution imaging of both the pancreatic parenchyma and ducts while simultaneously providing a means to sample the cyst and any associated solid components or enlarged peripancreatic lymph nodes (Samarasena et al. 2012). The ability of EUS imaging alone to distinguish mucinous from non-mucinous cysts is low [51 % (Brugge et al. 2004)], and interobserver variability among endosonographers for distinguishing neoplastic and nonneoplastic cysts is only fair [$\kappa=0.24$ (Ahmad et al. 2003)]. While certain imaging features can be very specific for IPMN such as identifying a clear connection of the cyst to the main pancreatic duct, imaging features alone are not able to grade a noninvasive IPMN.

EUS is performed using a linear echoendoscope with color Doppler to assess vascularity. To adequately drain cyst contents, a 22 G needle is typically used. For cysts >3 cm, or for those with particularly viscous fluid, a 19 G needle may be more effective. The needle is inserted into the lesion with an occluding stylet in place; the stylet is removed once the needle is in the cyst. The cyst contents are drained first, and then additional passes are made of any solid component. Despite the use of a stylet, gastrointestinal contamination may still be present in the aspirate sample, so wiping the outside of the needle prior to expressing the cyst contents into an empty vial or solid tissue in the needle onto a glass slide is advised.

Cyst fluid triage is discussed in the section below. Solid tissue expressed onto a glass slide requires knowledge of proper smear technique. The most cellular sample is useless if the cells are crushed, air-dried, or clotted in blood. A video of proper smearing technique can be found on the Papanicolaou Society of Cytopathology

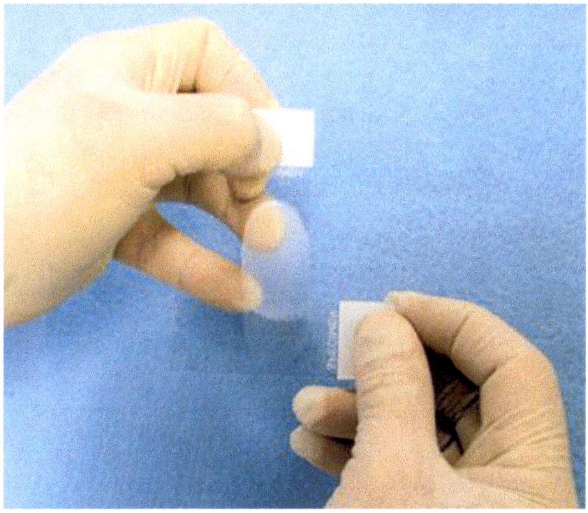

Fig. 7.1 Direct smearing technique. The aspirated tissue is expressed onto the glass slide near the label end, and a second glass slide is held perpendicular to the slide with the tissue to gently spread the cells down the slide

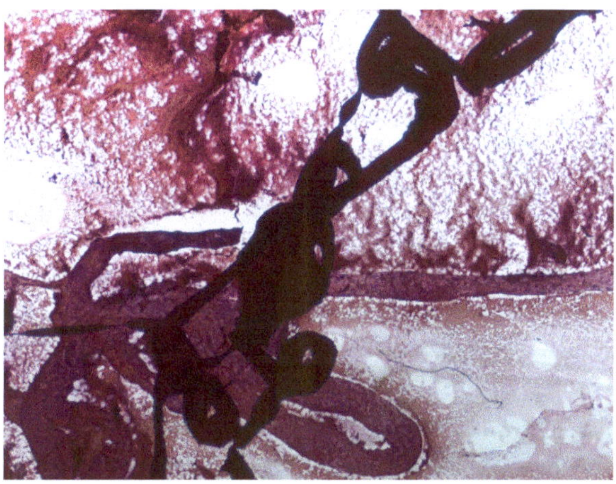

Fig. 7.2 Tissue trapped in blood. Tissue tends to clot if too much time is taken to express the tissue onto the glass slide. Entrapped tissue in blood clot cannot be interpreted and is a waste of tissue to keep on the slide (hematoxylin and eosin, ×40)

website (www.papsociey.org). In brief, the tissue is expressed onto the glass slide at the label end, and a second glass slide is held perpendicular to the slide with the tissue to gently spread the cells down the slide (Fig. 7.1). Slides can be fixed in alcohol or allowed to air-dry. Alcohol-stained smears provide the best nuclear detail. The smearing process should be performed quickly if the slide is to be fixed in alcohol to prevent air-drying artifact and blood clotting. Tissue trapped in blood clot is a waste of tissue and is useless to the pathologist; any "worm clots" (Fig. 7.2)

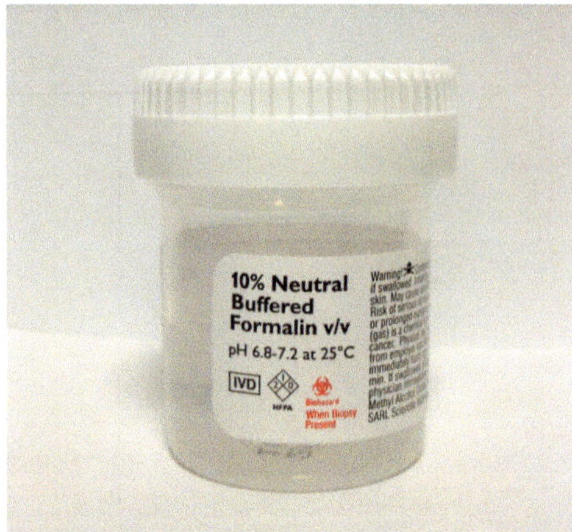

Fig. 7.3 Small container of 10 % neutral buffered formalin is useful for fixing tissue fragments and any tissue entrapped in blood clot as illustrated in Fig. 7.2

should be picked up off the slide with the needle tip and placed in a small formalin tub (e.g., the small tubs used for bone marrow biopsies) (Fig. 7.3).

Walsh et al. (2008) determined that a cyst size of 1.5 cm was needed to provide sufficient cyst fluid for at least one CFA test (cytology, CEA, or amylase) with an 84 % success rate.

7.1.1.1 Risks and Complications

The risk of EUS-FNA is low and generally limited to pancreatitis. In experienced centers, the complication rate is less than 1 % (Polkowski et al. 2012). Japanese investigators do not recommend EUS-FNA for the diagnosis of mucinous cystic lesions and believe that a cyst of any size with worrisome features should not be aspirated due to the risk of mucin spillage and the potential for peritoneal contamination during the biopsy (Hirooka et al. 2003; Yamao et al. 2011). However, a recent study from Massachusetts General Hospital of matched cohorts of patients with IPMN found that there was no difference in peritoneal seeding of cancer cells between the groups with or without preoperative EUS-FNA and there was no case of pseudomyxoma peritonei (Yoon et al. 2013). Given the shift toward conservative, nonsurgical management in a large percentage of patients with pancreatic cysts (Tanaka et al. 2012), the added value of CFA is important for early diagnosis of cancer.

7.2 Cyst Fluid Triage and Processing

7.2.1 Rapid On-Site Evaluation

The purpose of rapid on-site evaluation (ROSE) is to ensure that the FNA is adequately cellular for diagnosis and that the tissue aspirated is appropriately prepared and triaged for diagnosis. During the procedure, when the lesion is still available for additional sampling, is the time to evaluate the specimen for quality and cellular quantity. ROSE has been shown to be beneficial for solid mass lesions of the pancreas (Klapman et al. 2003; Iglesias-Garcia et al. 2011; Olson and Ali 2012), but no study has focused on the benefit of ROSE for pancreatic cysts. Generally, ROSE does not direct repeat biopsies of a cystic lesion. The cyst is drained until cyst collapse and the fluid is kept fresh for processing. If the cyst has a solid component, it is separately sampled with direct smears made for cytological analysis. ROSE requires a direct smear for immediate staining, and given that fluid specimens are typically often scant, the fluid should be appropriately triaged to ensure that the clinical questions regarding the cyst are specifically answered. Is the cyst mucinous? Is the cyst malignant?

7.2.1.1 Gross Inspection

The gross characteristics of the cyst fluid can be very informative, and these features should be recorded in the endoscopy note and relayed to the pathologist. A gross description such as "thick, white, viscous, sticky fluid" and cyst fluid that is difficult to pull into the needle and express from the needle clearly indicates a mucinous cyst fluid. These descriptions act as a surrogate marker for viscosity, a test that is not readily available in the biopsy suite. Leung et al. (2009) examined the role of the "string sign" as a marker of viscosity. By placing the fluid between the thumb and index finger and gently pulling the fingers apart, the fluid would "string" to 3.5 mm if mucinous. Ancillary testing adds little to this simple visual test. Fluid that is "thin and brown" or "thin and clear" may be mucinous or non-mucinous. CEA and amylase testing are very valuable in these circumstances.

The volume of cyst fluid is also important to record. The pathologist will note an obvious noncorrelation when only a "drop"' of fluid is obtained during aspiration and the slide is very cellular or covered with extracellular mucin or tissue. Such discordance should prompt the pathologist to consider gastrointestinal contamination or normal pancreatic tissue as the source of the tissue.

7.2.2 Triage of Cyst Fluid

Testing of cyst fluid is volume dependent. The quantity of aspirated cyst fluid varies widely, and for small branch-duct IPMN, cyst fluid may be extremely scant. If no visible cyst fluid is aspirated, then direct smears should be attempted from whatever tissue and fluid may be trapped in the needle and needle hub. Figure 7.4 outlines the cyst fluid triage protocol developed at the Massachusetts General Hospital. This triage protocol attempts to maximize high-yield information in an efficient and cost-effective way. Very small quantities of cyst fluid (<0.5 cc) are typically too scant in cellularity to make cytology a meaningful test. However, if imaging features are characteristic of an IPMN, then the remaining clinical question is whether there is cytological evidence of a high-grade lesion warranting resection. As such all of the

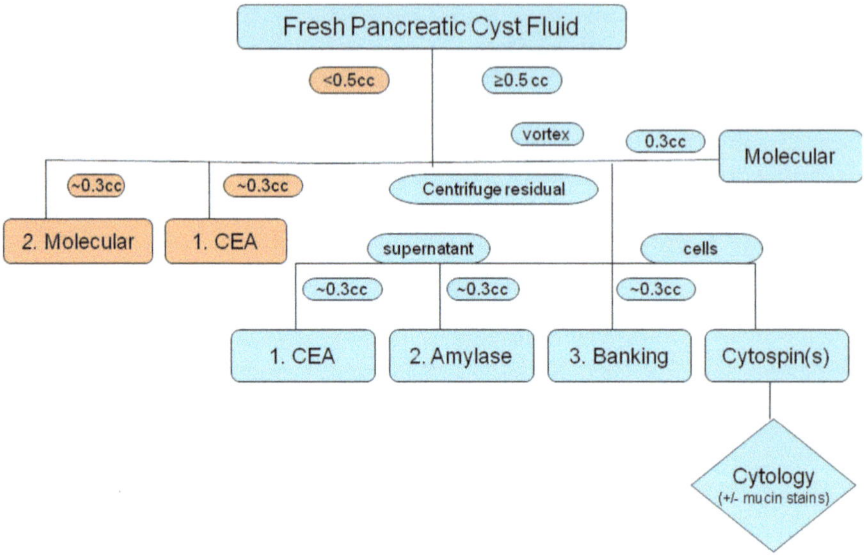

Fig. 7.4 Cyst fluid triage protocol developed at the Massachusetts General Hospital

cyst fluid should be sent for cytological analysis. If, however, the primary question is whether the cyst is mucinous or non-mucinous, for example, cyst aspirates <0.5 cc should be triaged to CEA or, if prior testing demonstrated a non-elevated CEA, molecular analysis.

Cyst fluids >0.5 cc offer sufficient volume for multiple ancillary tests. Cyst fluid should always remain fresh and unfixed and sent to the cytology lab for processing. An aliquot of neat fluid (~0.3 cc) is removed for molecular testing if needed and the remaining fluid is centrifuged. Although recent studies have shown that the supernatant fluid is rich in DNA (Chai et al. 2012), sufficient validation of this method remains to be determined. The cell button is processed as a cytospin(s) depending on the cellularity. Cytospins for mucin stains such as mucicarmine for neutral mucin and Alcian blue pH 2.5 for acid mucin can be performed. Since not all mucinous cysts in general or IPMNs in particular will demonstrate an elevation of CEA, and since thin mucin can be difficult to appreciate on cytology, mucin stains may be helpful (Fig. 7.5). Routine Papanicolaou staining of an alcohol-fixed cytospin allows for evaluation of nuclear detail. An air-dried cytospin may be stained with a Romanowsky stain such as Diff-Quik®, but nuclear detail is more difficult to evaluate with this stain. The supernatant fluid is then triaged to the chemistry lab for biochemical analysis.

The cell button can be reconstituted with preservatives such as Cytorich Red (Becton-Dickinson, Mountain Lake, NJ) or PreservCyt® (Hologic, Marlborough, MA) and processed as a ThinPrep or SurePath™ slide, respectively. The pathologist must keep in mind, however, that this method will significantly dilute the cyst fluid and attenuate extracellular mucin making it less easily recognized and distinguished from GI contamination.

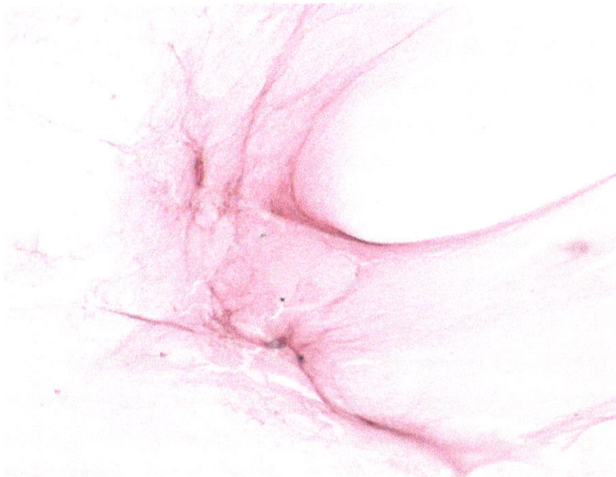

Fig. 7.5 Mucicarmine stain illustrating thin background mucin (×100)

7.3 Biochemical Analysis

7.3.1 Carcinoembryonic Antigen

In 2004, a multicenter prospective study showed that various combinations of cytological analysis and tumors markers, such as CA15-3, CA 19-9, CA 125, CA 72.4, and CEA, did not provide any additional diagnostic accuracy over CEA alone (Brugge et al. 2004). Since then, CEA has been shown to be the most reliable and accurate test for a mucinous cyst over mucin stains and cytology (Cizginer et al. 2011). Cutoff levels affect sensitivity and specificity. At a level of 192 ng/mL, CEA has an overall accuracy of ~80 % (specificity of 84 % and a sensitivity of 75 %) (Brugge et al. 2004). Raising the cutoff value improves specificity at the expense of sensitivity. At a level of 800 ng/mL, the specificity is 98 % but sensitivity is 48 % (van der Waaij et al. 2005). CEA levels also do not correlate with malignancy. Serous cystadenomas and pseudocysts typically have CEA levels <0.5 ng/mL. However, elevations of CEA may be seen in pseudocysts and other non-mucinous cysts, such as lymphoepithelial cysts (Raval et al. 2010), and nonneoplastic mucinous cysts such as gastrointestinal duplication cysts (Johnston et al. 2008). In addition, CEA is not always elevated in a mucinous cyst, so a low CEA level may be supportive of a non-mucinous cyst, but should not be interpreted as diagnostic of a non-mucinous cyst.

The measured CEA value of a patient's sample can vary depending on the testing procedure used, so each laboratory must validate the assay for normal and abnormal ranges. The CEA immunoassay uses the sandwich antibody method. CEA values determined on patient samples by different testing procedures cannot be directly compared with one another and could be the cause of erroneous medical interpretations.

7.3.2 *Amylase*

Amylase testing quantifies α-amylase using an enzymatic colorimetric assay to measure the formation of degradation products saccharogenically or kinetically with the aid of enzyme-catalyzed subsequent reactions. The color intensity of the degradation product formed is directly proportional to the α-amylase activity, which is determined by measuring the increase in absorbance.

The utility of amylase analysis in PCF is to support the clinical and cytological diagnosis of a pseudocyst or serous cystadenoma. Amylase levels are highly variable in mucinous cysts and do not distinguish between IPMN and MCN (Cizginer et al. 2011). Pseudocysts should always have a high amylase level, usually in the 1,000's due to the destruction of pancreatic acinar tissue; a low amylase level (<250 U/L) warrants clinical consideration of another diagnosis (van der Waaij et al. 2005).

7.4 Molecular Analysis

7.4.1 *KRAS and GNAS*

KRAS and *GNAS* mutations are assessed with polymerase chain reaction (PCR) of DNA from formalin-fixed paraffin-embedded tissue, aspirated cells by FNA, as well as from cyst or duct fluid, including supernatant fluid (Shi et al. 2008; Chai et al. 2012; Finkelstein et al. 2012). While the assessment of CEA is certainly a more cost-effective test to determine the mucinous nature of a cyst, not all mucinous cysts have an elevated CEA and an elevated CEA is not 100 % specific for a mucinous neoplasm.

Greater than 96 % of IPMNs have either a v-ki-ras2 Kirsten rat sarcoma (*KRAS*) or guanine nucleotide-binding protein alpha-stimulating, activity polypeptide 1 (*GNAS)* mutation, and more than half harbor both mutations (Wu et al. 2011). *KRAS* mutation is one of the earliest genetic mutations in pancreatic cancer with mutations predominantly occurring on codons 12 and 13 (Kitago et al. 2004). However, more than one mutant clone of *KRAS* may occur in a single IPMN cyst, and distinct IPMN cysts often have different *KRAS* mutations (Matthaei et al. 2012). *GNAS* mutations in PCF appear to occur only at codon 201, and this mutation seems to be specific to IPMNs and the invasive carcinomas arising from them (Furukawa et al. 2011; Wu et al. 2011). Using whole-exome sequencing of isolated DNA from IPMNs, Fukuwara et al. (2011) found mutations in 17 genes, including *GNAS*. The *GNAS* mutation, present in >40 % of IPMNs, was always at codon 201. The assessment of PCF for *GNAS* and other mutant genes by Wu et al. (2011) confirmed the presence of *GNAS* mutations in 66 % of IPMNs and the absence of them in MCN, serous cystadenomas, or solid-pseudopapillary neoplasms (SPNs). The detection of a

KRAS mutation supports the presence of a neoplastic mucinous cyst, and the detection of a *GNAS* mutation distinguishes an IPMN from an MCN. The value of testing for the *GNAS* mutation is particularly important when conservative management of a branch-duct IPMN is being considered and the distinction from other pancreatic cysts is not apparent from imaging studies or less expensive ancillary tests. Additionally, studies have shown that secretin-stimulated pancreatic juice harbors mutant *GNAS* in patients with IPMN and in patients who subsequently develop IPMNs suggesting that screening the pancreatic juice of patients at high-risk for pancreatic cancer may provide some risk stratification for subsequent surveillance(Kanda et al. 2012).

Unfortunately, these molecular markers are present in all grades of dysplasia, so the detection of neither mutant gene distinguishes a low-grade from high-grade mucinous cyst. In addition, the absence of both markers does not exclude a mucinous neoplasm.

7.4.2 Loss of Heterozygosity

The human genome is largely heterozygous. Loss of heterozygosity (LOH) is a common occurrence in cancers and indicates the absence of a functional tumor suppressor gene in the lost region either due to an absent or mutated allele. Although the identification of these regions has relied on genotyping tumor and normal DNA with recognition of regions where heterozygous alleles in the normal DNA become homozygous in the tumor, with the advent of oligonucleotide arrays that simultaneously assay thousands of single-nucleotide polymorphism (SNP) markers, genotyping can now be done at high enough resolution to allow identification of LOH without comparison to normal controls. In IPMN, the most frequent LOH occurs at chromosome 17q which involves the gene *RNF43* (Wu et al. 2011), a gene associated with E3 ubiquitin ligase activity (Sugiura et al. 2008). Some studies have suggested that the quality and quantity of DNA and the order in which *KRAS* mutations and LOH occur can distinguish benign from malignant IPMN (Khalid et al. 2005).

7.5 Potential Future Markers

Investigation into more sensitive and specific markers for the detection of mucinous and malignant cysts is intense. Several promising studies have looked at glycosylation variants of mucins (Haab et al. 2010), protein profiling (Shirai et al. 2008; Allen et al. 2009), and novel biomarkers such as plectin-1 (Bausch et al. 2009) and aberrant miRNAs (Ryu et al. 2011), but to date, none of these markers have been sufficiently validated for routine clinical use.

7.6 Cytological Analysis

Cytological analysis of pancreatic cyst fluid complements the biochemical and molecular analysis and is the most accurate test for the detection of malignancy (Cizginer et al. 2011). The limitations of cytological analysis rest with the scant and often degenerated nature of the cyst contents, the contamination of the aspirate with gastrointestinal mucosa and mucous, the lack of experience with the interpretation of this rare cytological specimen type outside of major medical centers, and finally, the nonstandardized terminology used to interpret these cytological specimens.

The cytological interpretation of PCF should not occur in a vacuum. A multimodal approach is required for an interpretation that is clinically useful (Pitman and Deshpande 2007). The (cyto)pathologist should review the report of the biopsy procedure and, in the case of EUS-FNA, should clearly understand the location of the cyst, the organ traversed during biopsy, and the amount of fluid aspirated. The cytological interpretation is greatly enhanced by reviewing any ancillary testing results so that these tests can be incorporated into the diagnosis to make for a more accurate and meaningful report.

It is important to understand the nomenclature of the classification of pancreatic cysts so that the cytological reports may be better understood. A cytological diagnosis often does not provide as specific a diagnosis as a histological diagnosis. Aspiration of cyst contents is not a directed biopsy of the cyst lining and wall. The aspiration of cyst contents is essentially a screening test for cancer, and the cells present in the cyst fluid may not represent the highest grade of dysplasia present in these typically heterogeneous cysts (Michaels et al. 2006).

The term "malignant" used to be rather straightforward because "carcinoma" was a part of the diagnostic nomenclature of both invasive and high-grade noninvasive cysts in the 2004 WHO classification of pancreatic cysts (Kloppel et al. 2000). The 2010 WHO classification system, however, distinguishes "malignant" and "premalignant" (Adsay et al. 2010) cysts by the presence of invasive carcinoma. As such, what used to be called "carcinoma in-situ" is now called "high-grade dysplasia," and what used to be called "borderline malignancy" is now called intermediate-grade (moderate) dysplasia. It can be extremely challenging to accurately cytologically distinguish the exact grade of cells that have exfoliated into the cyst fluid. As such, recommendations have been made to distinguish low-grade from high-grade epithelial atypia, the latter representing at least high-grade dysplasia with 85 % accuracy (Pitman et al. 2010).

7.6.1 Cytological Processing

It is optimal that the cytology lab receives all cyst fluids fresh for processing so that the lab can appropriately triage the fluid and be aware of all ancillary tests. The centrifuged cell button can be processed as a cytospin or reconstituted in proprietary

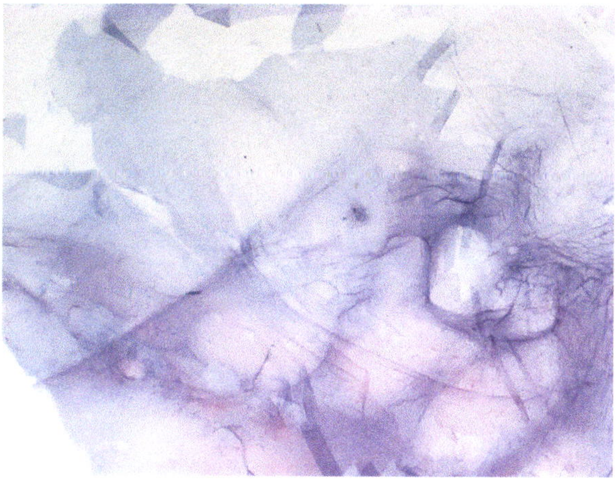

Fig. 7.6 Thick, colloid-like mucin is distinctive in quality and quantity from gastrointestinal mucin contamination and is indicative of a neoplastic mucinous cyst (Papanicolaou, ×200)

preservatives for liquid-based processing. Cytospins offer the most unaltered evaluation of the cells and cyst contents. Cytospins can be air-dried for Romanowsky stain, fixed in 95 % ethanol for Papanicolaou stain, and submitted for histochemical mucin stains or immunohistochemical stains such as synaptophysin in the case of a cystic neuroendocrine tumor.

7.6.2 Intraductal Papillary Mucinous Neoplasm

Aspirates of IPMN produce variable amounts of mucin and cyst-lining epithelium and, as such, may not accurately classify the cyst as mucinous, distinguish it as a mucinous cyst distinct from an MCN, or accurately grade the cyst due to the heterogeneity of the typical IPMN. A specific diagnosis of IPMN, therefore, is less common on FNA than a more general diagnosis of a neoplastic mucinous cyst, a term that encompasses both IPMN and MCN. This is primarily due to hypocellularity of the mucinous contents aspirated and a lack of architectural specificity of the glandular epithelium.

Thick and viscous typically white cyst fluid indicates mucin, which is reflected on the slide as "colloid-like" mucin (Fig. 7.6). Gastrointestinal mucin may appear focally thick but not "colloid-like." Degenerated inflammatory cells and histiocytes and stripped oval, grooved gastric epithelial naked nuclei within the mucin also help to distinguish cyst mucin from contaminating mucin. Thin mucin may be difficult to visualize on routine preparations and this is especially true on liquid-based preparations. This is where CEA or *KRAS* analysis is beneficial. Thin clear fluid without visible extracellular mucin, or thin mucin of uncertain origin and with an elevated

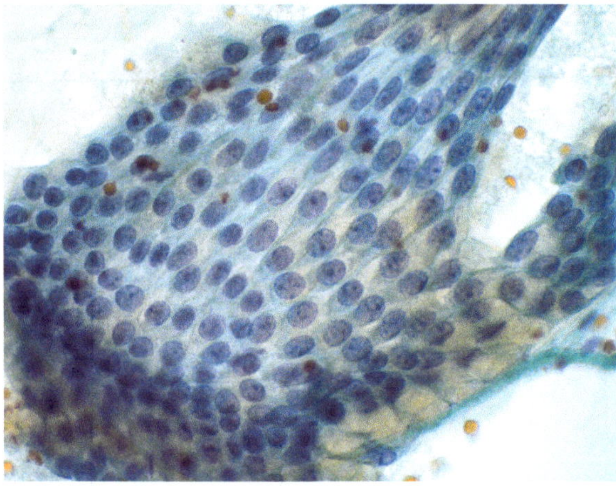

Fig. 7.7 Gastric foveolar epithelium presents as a uniform, geometric "honeycombed" sheet of epithelial cells with cytoplasmic mucin, which resembles low-grade dysplasia of the typical gastric-type lining of branch-duct IPMN (Papanicolaou; 600×)

CEA (>192 ng/mL at MGH), or a *KRAS* mutation, is consistent with a neoplastic mucinous cyst. Detection of a *GNAS* mutation supports the diagnosis of IPMN. Even if the cyst fluid is acellular and the grade of the cyst is unknown, the report can read "Acellular cyst fluid with elevated CEA [value] consistent with mucinous cyst" or "Acellular cyst fluid with *GNAS* mutation consistent with IPMN" rather than "non-diagnostic." A gastroenterologist or surgeon seeing this report in the context of low-risk imaging features of an IPMN is much better positioned to offer conservative management with the former report than the latter. A non-diagnostic cytology report may also lead to unnecessary repeat testing.

Evaluation of the cells in a cyst fluid has the primary goal of distinguishing low-grade-appearing epithelium from high-grade-appearing epithelium. Low-grade-appearing epithelium includes GI contamination, both gastric (Fig. 7.7) and duodenal (Fig. 7.8) mucosal contamination, normal pancreatic tissue, serous cystadenoma epithelium (Fig. 7.9), and low-grade mucinous epithelium (Fig. 7.10). High-grade-appearing epithelium includes adenocarcinoma (Fig. 7.11), high-grade dysplasia (Fig. 7.12), and (cystic) neuroendocrine tumor cells (Fig. 7.13). Although the cells of SPNs are bland and low-grade appearing, the shear volume of epithelium usually aspirated along with the classic solid and cystic imaging appearance makes this secondarily cystic neoplasm a rather straightforward diagnosis cytologically (Fig. 7.14).

IPMNs with low-grade dysplasia are lined by gastric foveolar-type cells that are impossible to accurately distinguish from gastric mucosal epithelial cells. The enterocytes of duodenal epithelial cells are non-mucinous except for the widely scattered goblet cells, so knowing that an EUS-FNA is transduodenal is very helpful to the pathologist in the interpretation of such cells. Low-grade dysplastic mucinous

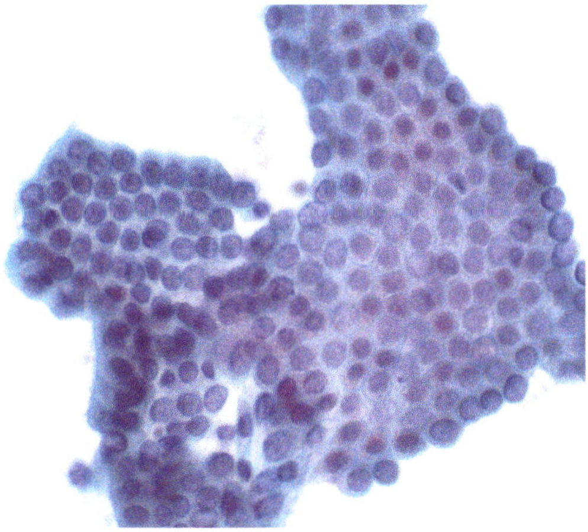

Fig. 7.8 Duodenal epithelium presents as a uniform, geometric "honeycombed" sheet of non-mucinous epithelial cells that have an apical brush border (Papanicolaou; 600×)

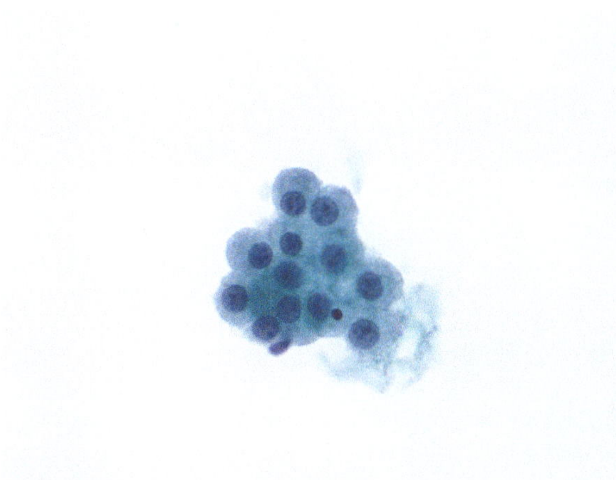

Fig. 7.9 Serous cystadenoma demonstrates bland cuboidal non-mucinous epithelial cells. (Papanicolaou; 600×)

epithelial cells are bland columnar mucinous glandular cells arranged in small clusters and flat to folded sheets with a honeycombed pattern. Single cells may also be seen. Mucinous papillary epithelial fragments are only rarely appreciated (see Fig. 7.10).

IPMNs with high-grade dysplasia contain cells with nuclear crowding, loss of polarity, nuclear elongation and hyperchromasia, irregular nuclear membranes, and high nuclear-to-cytoplasmic ratio. Cells may be arranged in papillary clusters where the length is usually twice the width of the group, small tight epithelial cells clusters,

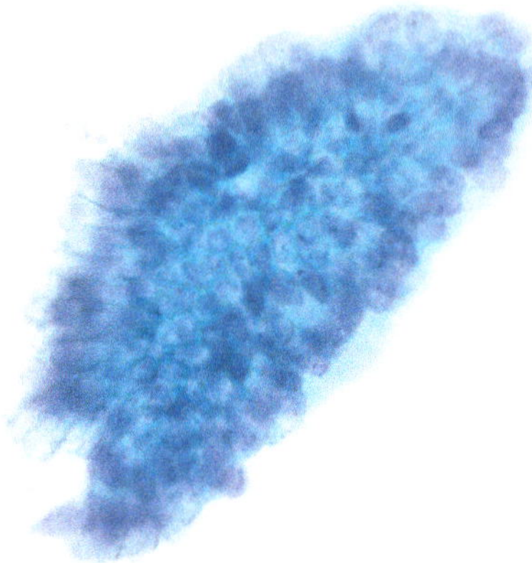

Fig. 7.10 IPMN with low-grade dysplasia resembles contaminating gastric epithelium with mucinous epithelial cells occasionally forming papillary groups. (Papanicolaou; 600×)

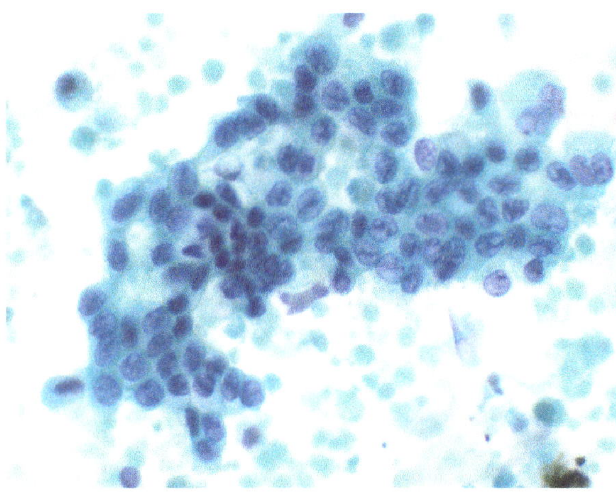

Fig. 7.11 Adenocarcinoma (invasive carcinoma) is recognized by cellular groups of cells with high nuclear to cytoplasmic ratio, abnormal chromatin and irregular nuclear membranes associated with background cellular necrosis (Papanicolaou; 600×)

or singly (see Fig. 7.12). Single dysplastic cells are smaller than the typical 12 micron duodenal enterocyte. Even if very scant in amount, the presence of cells with these features is significant (Pitman et al. 2010, in press) . Cellular hyperchromatic crowded groups of epithelial cells with open chromatin, thickened, irregular nuclear membranes and nucleoli with background cellular necrosis meet the cytological criteria for malignancy (see Fig. 7.13). IPMN with intermediate-grade dysplasia is very difficult to accurately classify as this grade of dysplasia includes gastric-type

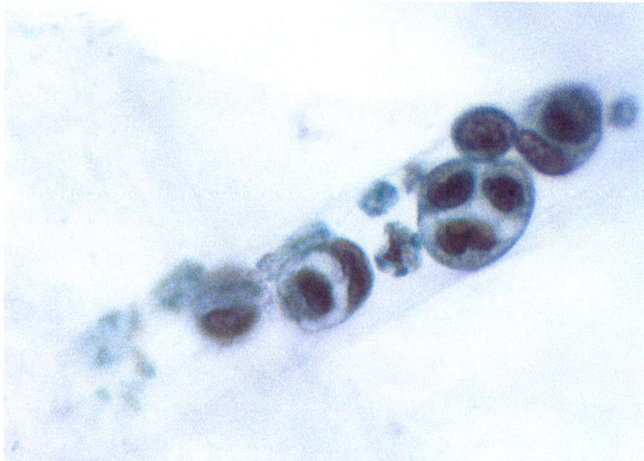

Fig. 7.12 High-grade dysplasia is often present only as single cells or small clusters with high nuclear to cytoplasmic ratio, abnormal chromatin and irregular nuclear membranes and no significant background cellular necrosis (Papanicolaou; 600×)

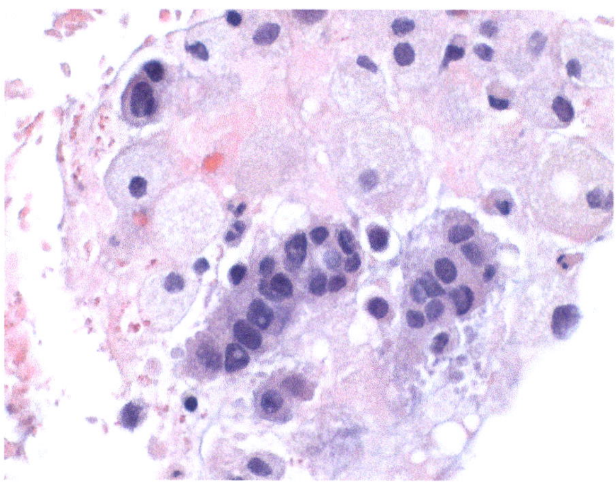

Fig. 7.13 Cystic neuroendocrine tumor produces high-grade appearing non-mucinous epithelial cells with coarse, stippled chromatin (Cellblock, Hematoxylin and eosin, ×600)

and intestinal-type epithelial cells. In an interobserver concordance study grading IPMN dysplasia, although intermediate-grade dysplasia was almost equally grouped in the low- and high-grade groups, it was best grouped in the low-grade category for highest accuracy (Pitman et al. in press). Although high-grade atypia may indeed represent some cases of intermediate- and low-grade dysplastic mucinous cysts as graded by histology, the recognition of such cells is a more sensitive indication for resection than imaging findings of a dilated main pancreatic duct or mural nodule (Genevay et al. 2011). The optimal time for resection of an IPMN with

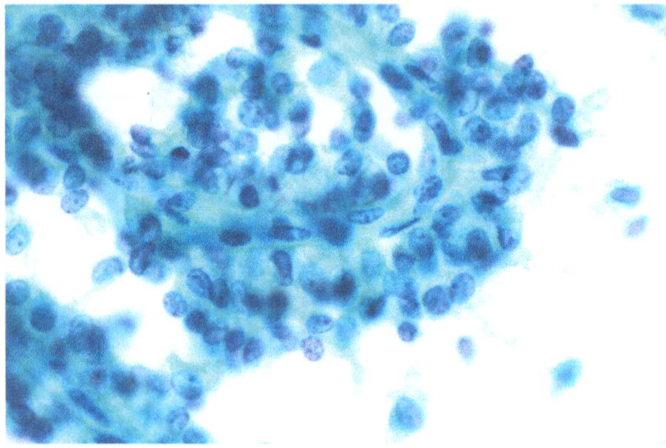

Fig. 7.14 Solid-pseudopapillary neoplasm typically produces very cellular smears with monomorphous cells containing relatively bland, grooved nuclei attached to vascular structures forming papillae, features that readily distinguish cyst from IPMN (Papanicolaou; 600×)

intermediate-grade dysplasia remains to be determined given the uncertainty of the time frame of the adenoma-carcinoma sequence. Ideally, only cysts with high-grade dysplasia would be resected providing the best prognosis with the lowest risk of operative morbidity. This ideal is unlikely to be met with the current screening tests at hand. With the pathologist part of the diagnostic team approach to patient care, an acceptable balance between sensitivity and specificity can be attained.

7.6.3 Differential Diagnosis

A differential diagnosis generally arises in the setting of a solitary branch-duct IPMN. The imaging features of main-duct and combined-type IPMN are rather straightforward, the latter when the connection between the branch-duct cyst and the main pancreatic duct is visualized. Also, multiple small cysts along the main pancreatic duct are a feature strongly supportive of branch-duct IPMN. The solitary cyst, however, has a broad differential diagnosis ranging from nonneoplastic lesions to malignancy. CFA is invaluable in the evaluation of these cysts, and it is the combination of clinical, imaging, biochemical, cytological, and molecular features that make the most accurate diagnosis.

Pseudocysts almost always occur in the setting of pancreatitis or abdominal trauma with abdominal pain. Alcohol abuse is a common etiological factor. EUS demonstrates a unilocular, nonseptated cyst with a thick cyst wall and typically internal debris. Cyst fluid is often brown and thin without viscosity (unless infected). Biochemical analysis invariably demonstrates a high amylase, usually in the thousands, and a low CEA; however, on rare occasions, CEA is elevated. A diagnosis of pseudocyst should not be made with low amylase (<250 ng/mL). Molecular analysis is negative. Cytological analysis reveals an inflammatory fluid with variable numbers of mixed inflammatory cells and histiocytes, yellow-hematoidin-like pigment, and no epithelial cells (Gonzalez 2009).

Serous cystadenomas are benign neoplasms that are usually asymptomatic but occasionally present with abdominal pain or palpable mass. Over 90 % demonstrate a lobulated, microcystic, honeycomb pattern on EUS; 10 % will be oligocystic or unilocular. Hypervascularity is commonly detected which correlates with high vascularity of the septa. Cyst fluid is often bloody but can be clear and should be thin and nonviscous. CEA and amylase levels are both low with CEA generally less than 5 ng/ml. Molecular analysis demonstrates either LOH or loss of 3p (VHL gene). Cytology is often disappointing and non-diagnostic due to the fragility of the cells. Hemosiderin-laden macrophages have been suggested as a surrogate marker (Belsley et al. 2008). The identification of non-mucinous cuboidal cells with clear (glycogen-rich) cytoplasm is consistent with serous epithelium (see Fig. 7.9).

Mucinous cystic neoplasms almost always occur in women, usually 40–50 years of age, and primarily in the body or tail of the gland. By definition these cysts are not connected to the main pancreatic duct. EUS demonstrates a unilocular or septated cyst that may have calcifications in the wall. The aspirate is mucinous with thick to thin extracellular mucin. CEA is often elevated above 192 ng/mL, but a level below that does not exclude a mucinous cyst. Amylase levels, although usually low, may be elevated, so a high amylase level does not distinguish IPMN from MCN. Molecular analysis shows *KRAS* mutations and mutations in *RNF43*; *GNAS* mutations are not present. Cytology alone does not distinguish IPMN from MCN in most cases; the ovarian-type stroma is not readily appreciated on the aspiration of cyst contents. The evaluation of epithelial atypia follows the same paradigm as for IPMN.

SPN is a secondarily cystic solid neoplasm that is not often confused with the other pancreatic cysts given its typically large, solid, and cystic imaging appearance, young patient age (20–30s), and almost exclusively female gender. FNAs do not usually aspirate fluid because the FNA target is the solid component. As such, CFA is not performed and smears are made of the very cellular aspirates, which depict numerous small, round to oval cells with a bland, uniform appearance. In addition to papillary fragments, tumor cell nuclei are bean shaped with grooves and the cytoplasm is scant and eccentric sometimes demonstrating perinuclear vacuoles or hyaline globules (see Fig. 7.14). Molecular analysis has demonstrated that *CTNNB1* is almost always mutated (Tanaka et al. 2001; Abraham et al. 2002). This mutation is associated with upregulation of beta-catenin, which is most cost-effectively detected by immunohistochemical stains showing nuclear staining.

Another solid, secondarily cystic neoplasm is pancreatic neuroendocrine tumor (cPanNET). In contrast to SPN, this cystic neoplasm is one that is often confused with primary pancreatic cysts. These cysts occur in men and women and can mimic both MCN and branch-duct IPMN. A clue on EUS is the very thick cyst wall. Aspirates more often produce cyst fluid. CEA and amylase levels are both low (Yoon et al. 2013). When epithelial cells are present, cytology is diagnostic given the characteristic endocrine features of the cells with round nuclei and coarse, stippled chromatin (see Fig. 7.13). Table 7.1 outlines the CFA features of these lesions.

Table 7.1 Gross, biochemical, molecular, and cytological characteristics of pancreatic cysts

	PCT	SCA	MCN	IPMN	SPN	cPanNET
Gross fluid						
Viscosity	↓	↓	↑↓	↑↓	↓	↓
Color	Brown	Clear Bloody	White Clear	White Clear	Bloody	Bloody
Biochemical						
CEA*	↓	↓	↑	↑	↓	↓
Amylase	↑↑	↓	↓↑	↑↓	↓	↓
Molecular						
KRAS	N	N	Y	Y	N	N
GNAS	N	N	N	Y	N	N
Others		*VHL (3p)*	*RNF43*	*RNF43*	*CTNNB1*	
Cytology						
ECM	N	N	Y	Y	N	N
Epithelial cells	None	Cuboidal	Mucinous	Mucinous	Non-mucinous	Endocrine
Atypia (grade)	NA	None	Low→high	Low→high	Low	Low→high
Background	Inflammatory Histiocytes Yellow pigment	Bloody Clear Hemosiderin-laden macrophages	Mucinous +/− cellular Necrotic debris	Mucinous +/− cellular Necrotic debris	Bloody +/− cellular Necrotic debris	Bloody +/− cellular Necrotic debris

PCT pseudocyst, *SCA* serous cystadenoma, *MCN* mucinous cystic neoplasm, *IPMN* intraductal papillary mucinous neoplasm, *SPN* solid-pseudopapillary neoplasm; *cPanNET* cystic pancreatic neuroendocrine tumor, *CEA* carcinoembryonic antigen, *VEGF* vascular endothelial growth factor, *ECM* extracellular mucin
*relative to 192 ng/ml

References

Abraham SC, Klimstra DS, et al. Solid-pseudopapillary tumors of the pancreas are genetically distinct from pancreatic ductal adenocarcinomas and almost always harbor beta-catenin mutations. Am J Pathol. 2002;160(4):1361–9.

Adsay NV, Fukushima N, et al. Intraductal neoplasms of the pancreas. In: Bosman FT, Carneiro F, Hruban RH, Theise ND, editors. WHO classification of tumours of the digestive system. France: IARC; 2010. p. 304–13.

Ahmad NA, Kochman ML, et al. Interobserver agreement among endosonographers for the diagnosis of neoplastic versus non-neoplastic pancreatic cystic lesions. Gastrointest Endosc. 2003; 58(1):59–64.

Allen PJ, Qin LX, et al. Pancreatic cyst fluid protein expression profiling for discriminating between serous cystadenoma and intraductal papillary mucinous neoplasm. Ann Surg. 2009;250(5):754–60.

Alles AJ, Warshaw AL, et al. Expression of CA 72–4 (TAG-72) in the fluid contents of pancreatic cysts. A new marker to distinguish malignant pancreatic cystic tumors from benign neoplasms and pseudocysts. Ann Surg. 1994;219(2):131–4.

Bausch D, Mino-Kenudson M, et al. Plectin-1 is a biomarker of malignant pancreatic intraductal papillary mucinous neoplasms. J Gastrointest Surg. 2009;13(11):1948–54. discussion 1954.

Belsley NA, Pitman MB, et al. Serous cystadenoma of the pancreas: limitations and pitfalls of endoscopic ultrasound-guided fine-needle aspiration biopsy. Cancer. 2008;114(2):102–10.

Brugge WR, Lewandrowski K, et al. Diagnosis of pancreatic cystic neoplasms: a report of the cooperative pancreatic cyst study. Gastroenterology. 2004;126(5):1330–6.

Chai SM, Herba K, et al. Optimizing the multimodal approach to pancreatic cyst fluid diagnosis: developing a volume based triage protocol. Cancer Cytopathol. 2012;121:86–100.

Cizginer S, Turner B, et al. Cyst fluid carcinoembryonic antigen is an accurate diagnostic marker of pancreatic mucinous cysts. Pancreas. 2011;40(7):1024–8.

Finkelstein SD, Bibbo M, et al. Molecular analysis of centrifugation supernatant fluid from pancreaticobiliary duct samples can improve cancer detection. Acta Cytol. 2012;56(4):439–47.

Furukawa T, Kuboki Y, et al. Whole-exome sequencing uncovers frequent GNAS mutations in intraductal papillary mucinous neoplasms of the pancreas. Sci Rep. 2011;1:161.

Genevay M, Mino-Kenudson M, et al. Cytology adds value to imaging studies for risk assessment of malignancy in pancreatic mucinous cysts. Ann Surg. 2011;254(6):977–83.

Gonzalez Obeso E, Murphy E, et al. Pseudocyst of the pancreas. Cancer Cytopathol. 2009;117: 101–7.

Haab BB, Porter A, et al. Glycosylation variants of mucins and CEACAMs as candidate biomarkers for the diagnosis of pancreatic cystic neoplasms. Ann Surg. 2010;251(5):937–45.

Hammel P, Levy P, et al. Preoperative cyst fluid analysis is useful for the differential diagnosis of cystic lesions of the pancreas. Gastroenterology. 1995;108(4):1230–5.

Hirooka Y, Goto H, et al. Case of intraductal papillary mucinous tumor in which endosonography-guided fine-needle aspiration biopsy caused dissemination. J Gastroenterol Hepatol. 2003; 18(11):1323–4.

Iglesias-Garcia J, Dominguez-Munoz JE, et al. Influence of on-site cytopathology evaluation on the diagnostic accuracy of endoscopic ultrasound-guided fine needle aspiration (EUS-FNA) of solid pancreatic masses. Am J Gastroenterol. 2011;106(9):1705–10.

Johnston J, Wheatley 3rd GH, et al. Gastric duplication cysts expressing carcinoembryonic antigen mimicking cystic pancreatic neoplasms in two adults. Am Surg. 2008;74(1):91–4.

Kanda M, Knight S, et al. Mutant GNAS detected in duodenal collections of secretin-stimulated pancreatic juice indicates the presence or emergence of pancreatic cysts. Gut. 2012;62:1024–33.

Khalid A, McGrath KM, et al. The role of pancreatic cyst fluid molecular analysis in predicting cyst pathology. Clin Gastroenterol Hepatol. 2005;3(10):967–73.

Khalid A, Zahid M, et al. Pancreatic cyst fluid DNA analysis in evaluating pancreatic cysts: a report of the PANDA study. Gastrointest Endosc. 2009;69(6):1095–102.

Kitago M, Ueda M, et al. Comparison of K-ras point mutation distributions in intraductal papillary-mucinous tumors and ductal adenocarcinoma of the pancreas. Int J Cancer. 2004;110(2):177–82.

Klapman JB, Logrono R, et al. Clinical impact of on-site cytopathology interpretation on endoscopic ultrasound-guided fine needle aspiration. Am J Gastroenterol. 2003;98(6):1289–94.

Kloppel G, Hruban RH, et al. Tumours of the exocrine pancreas. In: Hamilton SR, Aaltonen LA, editors. WHO classification of tumours- pathology and genetics of tumours of the digestive system. Lyon: IARC press; 2000. p. 219–30.

Leung KK, Ross WA, et al. Pancreatic cystic neoplasm: the role of cyst morphology, cyst fluid analysis, and expectant management. Ann Surg Oncol. 2009;16(10):2818–24.

Lewandrowski K, Warshaw A, et al. Macrocystic serous cystadenoma of the pancreas. Hum Pathol. 1992;23:871–5.

Lewandrowski K, Lee J, et al. Cyst fluid analysis in the differential diagnosis of pancreatic cysts: a new approach to the preoperative assessment of pancreatic cystic lesions. AJR. 1995;164:815–9.

Matthaei H, Norris AL, et al. Clinicopathological characteristics and molecular analyses of multifocal intraductal papillary mucinous neoplasms of the pancreas. Ann Surg. 2012;255(2):326–33.

Michaels PJ, Brachtel EF, et al. Intraductal papillary mucinous neoplasm (IPMN) of the pancreas: cytohistologic analysis and correlation with histologic grade. Cancer Cytopathol. 2006;108(3): 163–73.

Olson MT, Ali SZ. Cytotechnologist on-site evaluation of pancreas fine needle aspiration adequacy: comparison with cytopathologists and correlation with the final interpretation. Acta Cytol. 2012;56(4):340–6.

Pitman MB, Centeno BA, Daglilar ES, et al. Cytological Criteria of High-Grade Epithelial Atypia in the Cyst Fluid of Pancreatic Intraductal Papillary Mucinous Neoplasms. Cancer Cytopathol. (in press)

Pitman MB, Centeno B, Genevay M, et al. Grading Epithelial Atypia in EUS-FNA of Pancreatic Mucinous Cysts: An International Interobserver Concordance Study. Cancer Cytopathol. (in press)

Pitman MB, Deshpande V. Endoscopic ultrasound-guided fine needle aspiration cytology of the pancreas: a morphological and multimodal approach to the diagnosis of solid and cystic mass lesions. Cytopathology. 2007;18(6):331–47.

Pitman MB, Genevay M, et al. High-grade atypical epithelial cells in pancreatic mucinous cysts are a more accurate predictor of malignancy than "positive" cytology. Cancer Cytopathol. 2010;118:434–40.

Polkowski M, Larghi A, et al. Learning, techniques, and complications of endoscopic ultrasound (EUS)-guided sampling in gastroenterology: European society of gastrointestinal endoscopy (ESGE) technical guideline. Endoscopy. 2012;44(2):190–206.

Raval JS, Zeh HJ, et al. Pancreatic lymphoepithelial cysts express CEA and can contain mucous cells: potential pitfalls in the preoperative diagnosis. Mod Pathol. 2010;23(11):1467–76.

Rubin D, Warshaw AL, et al. Expression of CA 15.3 protein in the cyst contents distinguishes benign from malignant pancreatic mucinous cystic neoplasms. Surgery. 1994;115(1):52–5.

Ryu JK, Matthaei H, et al. Elevated microRNA miR-21 levels in pancreatic cyst fluid are predictive of mucinous precursor lesions of ductal adenocarcinoma. Pancreatology. 2011;11(3):343–50.

Samarasena JB, Nakai Y, et al. Endoscopic ultrasonography-guided fine-needle aspiration of pancreatic cystic lesions: a practical approach to diagnosis and management. Gastrointest Endosc Clin N Am. 2012;22(2):169–85. vii.

Shi C, Fukushima N, et al. Sensitive and quantitative detection of KRAS2 gene mutations in pancreatic duct juice differentiates patients with pancreatic cancer from chronic pancreatitis, potential for early detection. Cancer Biol Ther. 2008;7(3):353–60.

Shirai Y, Sogawa K, et al. Protein profiling in pancreatic juice for detection of intraductal papillary mucinous neoplasm of the pancreas. Hepatogastroenterology. 2008;55(86–87):1824–9.

Sugiura T, Yamaguchi A, et al. A cancer-associated RING finger protein, RNF43, is a ubiquitin ligase that interacts with a nuclear protein, HAP95. Exp Cell Res. 2008;314(7):1519–28.

Tanaka Y, Kato K, et al. Frequent beta-catenin mutation and cytoplasmic/nuclear accumulation in pancreatic solid-pseudopapillary neoplasm. Cancer Res. 2001;61(23):8401–4.

Tanaka M, Fernandez-del Castillo C, et al. International consensus guidelines 2012 for the management of IPMN and MCN of the pancreas. Pancreatology. 2012;12(3):183–97.

Tatsuta M, Iishi H, et al. Values of carcinoembryonic antigen, elastase 1, and carbohydrate antigen determinant in aspirated pancreatic cystic fluid in the diagnosis of cysts of the pancreas. Cancer. 1986;57(9):1836–9.

van der Waaij LA, van Dullemen HM, et al. Cyst fluid analysis in the differential diagnosis of pancreatic cystic lesions: a pooled analysis. Gastrointest Endosc. 2005;62(3):383–9.

Walsh RM, Vogt DP, et al. Management of suspected pancreatic cystic neoplasms based on cyst size. Surgery. 2008;144(4):677–84. discussion 684–675.

Wu J, Matthaei H, et al. Recurrent GNAS mutations define an unexpected pathway for pancreatic cyst development. Sci Transl Med. 2011;3(92):92ra66.

Wu RW, Yoon J, et al. Endoscopic ultrasound-guided fine needle aspiration (EUS-FNA) contributes to a triple negative test in preoperative screening of pancreatic cysts. J Am Soc Cytopathol. 2012;1 Suppl 103:186-A.

Yamao K, Yanagisawa A, et al. Clinicopathological features and prognosis of mucinous cystic neoplasm with ovarian-type stroma: a multi-institutional study of the Japan pancreas society. Pancreas. 2011;40(1):67–71.

Yoon WJ, Dagilar ES, et al. Peritoneal Seeding in Intraductal Papillary Mucinous Neoplasm of the Pancreas Patients WHO Underwent Endoscopic Ultrasound-Guided Fine-Needle Aspiration; Results of the PIPE Study. Gastrointest Endosc. 2013; 77 (Supp:5) AB409.

Chapter 8
Diagnostic Investigation Using Pancreatic Juice

Takao Ohtsuka, Fumihiko Ookubo, and Masao Tanaka

Abstract Although endoscopic retrograde pancreatography to collect pancreatic juice sample for intraductal papillary mucinous neoplasms (IPMNs) of the pancreas is not routinely recommended because of its possible severe complication of pancreatitis, assessments of cytology and molecular markers in pancreatic juice are often useful to diagnose malignant IPMNs. In addition, pancreatic juice cytology is the only way to detect early stage pancreatic ductal adenocarcinoma concomitant with IPMNs which cannot be detected by imaging modalities such as computed tomography, magnetic resonance imaging, or endoscopic ultrasonography. The sensitivity of pancreatic juice cytology for malignant IPMNs is not high, ranging from 10 % to 50 %; however, several molecular markers in pancreatic juice such as carcinoembryonic antigen level, MUC1 level, and the activity of telomerase improve the sensitivity. Pancreatic juice cytology also provides the information regarding subtypes of IPMNs, namely, gastric, intestinal, pancreatobiliary, and oncocytic by the assessments of morphological features and immunohistochemistry. On the other hand, it remains unclear which patients with IPMN are indication for pancreatic juice assessment and which patients really get benefits of such investigation.

Keywords Cytology • IPMN • Molecular marker • Pancreatic juice

---

T. Ohtsuka (✉) • M. Tanaka
Department of Surgery and Oncology, Graduate School of Medical Sciences, Kyushu University, Fukuoka, Japan
e-mail: takao-o@med.kyushu-u.ac.jp

F. Ookubo
Division of Diagnostic Pathology, Kyushu University Hospital, Fukuoka, Japan

M. Tanaka (ed.), *Intraductal Papillary Mucinous Neoplasm of the Pancreas*,
DOI 10.1007/978-4-431-54472-2_8, © Springer Japan 2014

8.1 Methods for Collecting Pancreatic Juice

Aspiration of the pancreatic juice through the catheter in the pancreatic duct under the endoscopic retrograde pancreatography (ERP) is the most popular method to collect pancreatic juice. Direct insertion of the catheter into the branch duct IPMN (BD-IPMN) is sometimes possible to collect cystic fluid; however, it is difficult in most cases of asymptomatic small BD-IPMNs. Another possible way is to aspirate the pancreatic juice under the endoscopic ultrasonography-guided fine needle aspiration (EUS-FNA) technique; however, it will be indicated for only limited cases. EUS-FNA during the assessment of IPMNs is basically performed for the collection of cystic fluid, and details in this issue are described in another chapter (Chap. 7). Duodenal juice includes pancreatic juice and the assessment of duodenal juice collected by duodenoscope or regular upper gastrointestinal scope is often useful to diagnose IPMNs by molecular analyses of *GNAS* mutation (Kanda et al. 2013) or protein levels of carcinoembryonic antigen (CEA) and S100 (Mori et al. 2013). Although collection of the duodenal juice is less invasive and easier than the pancreatic juice aspiration under ERP, cytological assessment of duodenal juice seems to be difficult and it still remains unclear whether the assessment of duodenal juice always reflects the component of pancreatic juice.

8.2 Endoscopic Retrograde Pancreatography

EUS-FNA has recently taken the place of ERP in terms of cytological confirmation of various pancreatic diseases, and EUS-FNA technique can directly aspirate the cystic fluid of IPMN for the cytological assessment as well as related molecular analyses (Salla et al. 2007; Marie et al. 2008; Kucera et al. 2012). On the other hand, EUS-FNA has a risk of later peritoneal dissemination or needle tract seeding in the cases of malignant IPMNs and can assess only the limited area in the cases of multifocal BD-IPMNs (Paquin et al. 2005; Ahmed et al. 2011; Chong et al. 2011; Katanuma et al. 2012).

Although ERP for the collection of pancreatic juice is not routinely recommended during the management of BD-IPMNs in international consensus guidelines 2012 (Tanaka et al. 2012) because of its possible severe complication of pancreatitis, ERP still has important roles in the assessment of IPMNs. Dilated orifice of the duodenal papilla by the hypersecretion of mucin, presence of the mucin in the pancreatic duct, and communication between dilated cystic duct and main pancreatic duct detected by pancreatography are the direct evidences of the presence of IPMNs (Tanaka et al. 2012). ERP-guided intraductal ultrasonography and baby-scope assessments of main pancreatic duct are also useful to observe the spread of the lesions as well as to determine the resection line during pancreatectomy, especially in main duct IPMNs (MD-IPMNs) (Yamaguchi et al. 2005b). In addition, recent report has shown that pancreatic juice cytology under ERP is the only way to diagnose early stage pancreatic ductal adenocarcinomas (PDACs) concomitant with IPMNs, which cannot be detected by other imaging modalities such

Table 8.1 Summary of the issues regarding investigation using pancreatic juice during management of IPMNs

1. Endoscopic retrograde pancreatography for the collection of pancreatic juice in patients with IPMNs is not routinely recommended in international consensus guidelines 2012
2. Sensitivity of pancreatic juice cytology to detect malignant IPMN is reported to be 10–50 %
3. Potential molecular markers in pancreatic juice to increase the diagnostic ability for malignant IPMNs: carcinoembryonic antigen (CEA), MUC1, telomerase activity, etc.
4. Morphological subtype of IPMNs can be classified using preoperative pancreatic juice samples with 79 % of agreement
5. Pancreatic juice cytology is the only way to detect early stage pancreatic ductal adenocarcinoma concomitant with IPMNs which cannot be detected by imaging modalities
6. Intraoperative pancreatic juice cytology is useful to diagnose the presence of the unexpected lesions during pancreatectomy for IPMN

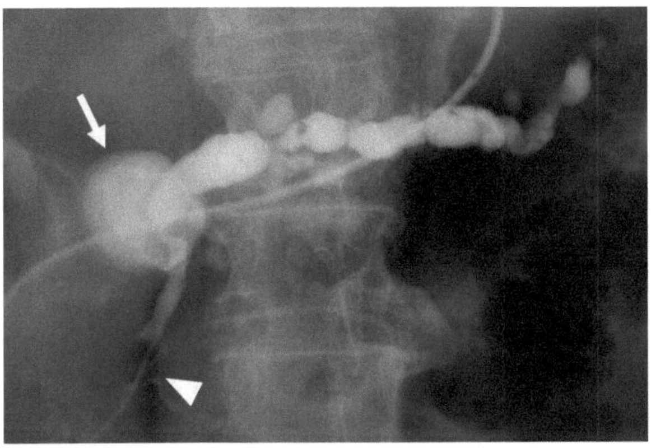

Fig. 8.1 Endoscopic retrograde pancreatography using balloon catheter. Balloon catheter (6Fr) is put into the main pancreatic duct, and the balloon is inflated near the duodenal papilla (*arrow head*). Then, the endoscope is withdrawn, leaving the balloon catheter in place. Pancreatography reveals cystic dilation of branch duct, 30 mm in diameter, in the head of the pancreas (*arrow*) and dilation of the upstream of the main pancreatic duct. After pancreatography, pancreatic juice is collected through balloon catheter under the secretin administration

as computed tomography (CT), magnetic resonance imaging (MRI), or endoscopic ultrasonography (EUS) (Ohtsuka et al. 2013). Several reports also demonstrated the utility of molecular assessment of pancreatic juice for the diagnosis of malignant IPMNs and subtype classification of IPMNs (Inoue et al. 2001; Hibi et al. 2007; Hirono et al. 2009; Mizuno et al. 2010; Shimamoto et al. 2010; Hirono et al. 2012). The issues regarding investigation using pancreatic juice during management of IPMNs are summarized in Table 8.1.

To fulfill the pancreatic ductal system by contrast medium for the assessment of IPMNs and subsequently to collect the pancreatic juice efficiently, balloon catheter put in the main pancreatic duct near the duodenal papilla is useful to prevent the leakage of pancreatic juice into the duodenum (Yamaguchi et al. 2005a) (Fig. 8.1). For the collection of enough amount of pancreatic juice, secretin administration is usually helpful (Yamaguchi et al. 2005a; Hibi et al. 2007).

8.2.1 Cytology

The sensitivity of pancreatic juice cytology to detect malignant IPMN including carcinoma in situ (high-grade dysplasia) and invasive carcinoma seems not to be high, ranging from 10 % to 50 % (Yamaguchi et al. 2005a, b; Hibi et al. 2007; Hirono et al. 2012). There are several factors influencing the sensitivity of pancreatic juice cytology: the distance from the duodenal papilla (pancreas head or body to tail), tumor location (MD- or BD-IPMN), pancreatic exocrine function (amount of collected pancreatic juice), and viscosity of pancreatic juice (mucin rich or not) (Yamaguchi et al. 2005a).

The sensitivity of pancreatic juice cytology of the IPMN is expected to be higher in the proximal pancreas than that in the distal pancreas; however, this parameter does not influence to the result of cytology (Yamaguchi et al. 2005b). We can easily access the dilated main pancreatic duct of MD-IPMN and directly correct the fluid of the tumor rather than BD-IPMN, and in fact, sensitivity of pancreatic juice cytology for malignant MD-IPMN has been reported to be higher than that of BD-IPMN (Yamaguchi et al. 2005a, b). High viscosity of pancreatic juice by mucin leads to difficulty in collection of the pancreatic juice through regular thin ERP catheter. Instead, aspiration through thick catheter or large working channel of the baby scope increases the amount of aspirated pancreatic juice and results in the improvement of the sensitivity to diagnose malignant IPMN (Yamaguchi et al. 2005b) (Fig. 8.2). Baby scope also provides a direct visualization of the lesion and an opportunity of biopsy (Yamaguchi et al. 2005b; Judah and Draganov 2008).

If the pancreatic juice cytology demonstrates positive result despite the imaging studies show benign-looking BD-IPMN, the possible presence of concomitant PDAC should be considered (Yamaguchi et al. 2005a). If the concomitant PDAC is noninvasive, then it is difficult to determine the location of the lesion. In this case, pancreatic juice cytology under segmental balloon ERP (Tanaka et al 1997) or intraoperative irrigation cytology of pancreatic duct is helpful (Mori et al 2010).

Cytological assessment for malignant IPMN is usually difficult even in the experienced pathologist or cytologist, because malignant IPMNs have well-differentiated structure and different dysplastic area even in one lesion ranging from low-, intermediate-, and high-grade dysplasia to invasive carcinoma (Yamaguchi et al. 2005a). Unfortunately, we still often experience the false-positive or false-negative results of pancreatic juice cytology during management of IPMNs.

8.2.2 Assessment of Malignant IPMNs

For the improvement of the sensitivity to diagnose malignant IPMN, several molecular markers in pancreatic juice have been validated. Hirono et al. (2012) have recently reported that CEA level in pancreatic juice over 30 ng/mL in addition to the size of mural nodule over 5 mm is a good predictor for malignant BD-IPMNs, of

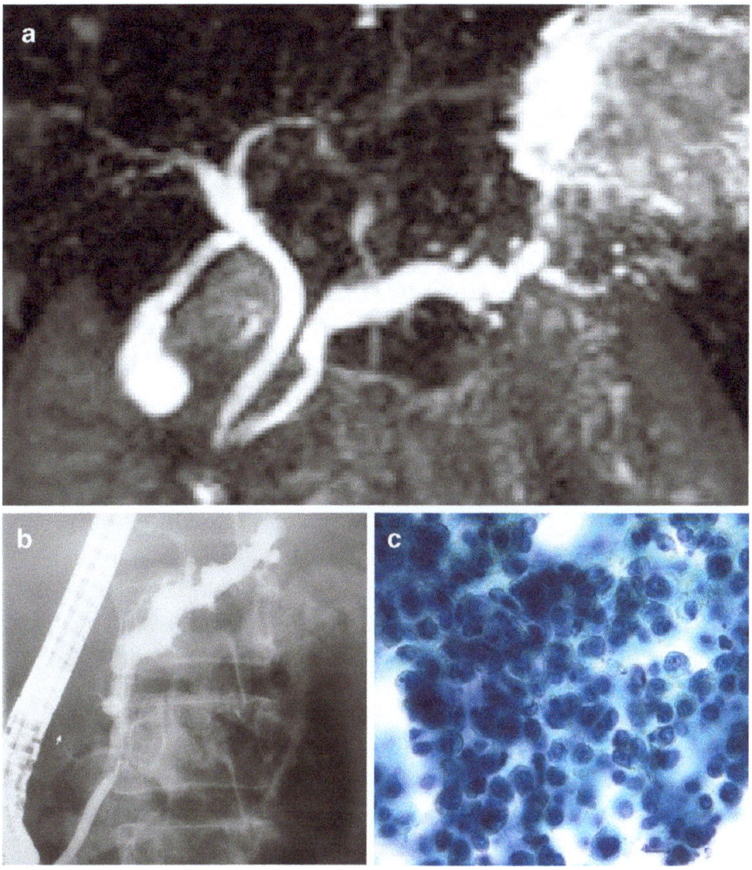

Fig. 8.2 Pancreatic juice cytology using baby scope. (**a**) Magnetic resonance cholangiopancreatography demonstrates the dilation of main pancreatic duct in the pancreatic body to tail, indicating main duct IPMN. (**b**) Endoscopic retrograde pancreatography (ERP) using baby scope, SpyGlass system (Boston Scientific, Natick, MA, USA). (**c**) Pancreatic juice cytology using SpyGlass system shows adenocarcinoma. In this patient, adenocarcinoma could not be detected by pancreatic juice cytology using regular ERP catheter, while SpyGlass system allows collecting much amount of pancreatic juice through large working channel

which positive and negative predictive value are 100 % and 96.3 %, respectively. This group also showed that CEA level in pancreatic juice over 110 ng/mL could predict malignant IPMNs including both branch duct and main duct types (Hirono et al. 2009). The reason for lower cutoff value of CEA in pancreatic juice in BD-IPMNs is considered that pancreatic juice collected from MD-IPMNs has larger amount of secreted mucin from neoplastic cells than BD-IPMNs, and secreted CEA from BD-IPMNs might be diluted with normal pancreatic juice.

Shimamoto et al. (2010) have shown that high MUC1 mRNA level in pure pancreatic juice collected by ERP is a useful marker for malignant IPMNs. When the cutoff value of MUC1 ratio to glyceraldehyde-3-phosphate dehydrogenase mRNA is set at 1,600, the sensitivity, specificity, and accuracy for malignant IPMNs are 88.9 %, 71.4 %, and 81.3 %, respectively. Inoue et al. (2001) demonstrated that high telomerase activity in pancreatic juice increased the sensitivity for the detection of malignant IPMN to 85 %, when comparing 31 % of the sensitivity of pancreatic juice cytology only.

8.2.3 Assessment of Subtype of IPMNs

IPMNs are pathologically classified into 4 subtypes, namely, gastric, intestinal, pancreatobiliary, and oncocytic (Furukawa et al 2005). The majority of IPMNs have gastric or intestinal subtype, and pancreatobiliary and oncocytic are rare subtypes, both of which are usually of malignant IPMNs. Most of IPMNs with gastric subtype have benign character, while IPMNs with intestinal subtype have high prevalence of malignancy but favorable prognosis after resection (Sohn et al. 2004; Poultsides et al. 2010; Sadakari et al. 2010; Furukawa et al. 2011; Mino-Kenudson et al. 2011; Yopp et al. 2011). Thus, preoperative diagnosis of intestinal subtype of IPMNs will lead to strong recommendation of the resection. In fact, classification of morphological subtype of IPMNs can be determined using pancreatic juice samples with 79 % of agreement between cytological and pathological assessments (Hibi et al. 2007) (Fig. 8.3). Intestinal subtype of IPMN is characterized as expression of MUC2 (Furukawa et al. 2005), and therefore, analyses of MUC2 protein expression by immunohistochemistry using pancreatic juice sample (Fig. 8.4) or MUC2 mRNA level in pancreatic juice by quantitative reverse transcriptional polymerase chain reaction (qRT-PCR) might support the morphological classification during cytological assessment (Tanaka et al. 2012).

8.2.4 Other Molecular Assessments

Several investigators have made efforts to assess the molecular markers in pancreatic juice to diagnose IPMNs or to predict malignant IPMNs. The most frequent mutation site of *KRAS* is at codon 12, and Kondo et al. (1997) demonstrates that 92 % of the patients with IPMNs had *KRAS* mutation by the assessment of pancreatic juice; however, *KRAS* mutation status could not distinguish malignant IPMNs from benign. This should be true because *KRAS* mutation is the early event during the progression of IPMNs, and Kaino et al. (1999) have shown the high frequency of *KRAS* mutation even in benign IPMNs using resected specimens. On the other hand, Mizuno et al. (2010) focused on the 6 different clonal patterns of *KRAS* mutations at codon 12 and found that single-clonal convergence of *KRAS* mutation was associated with malignant progression of IPMNs.

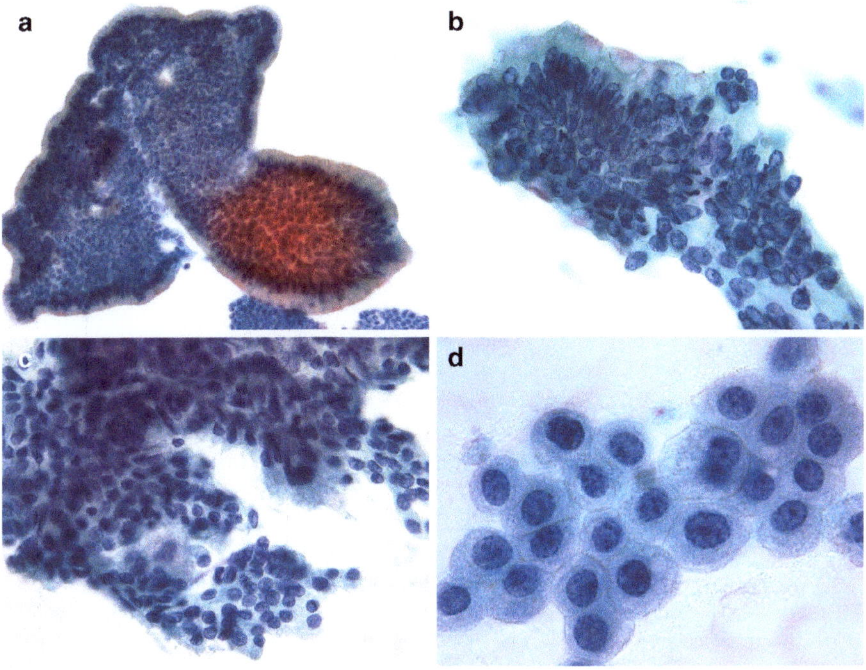

Fig. 8.3 Diagnosis of morphological subtypes of IPMNs using pancreatic juice samples. (**a**) Gastric subtype with mild atypia. Neoplastic cells are arranged in dense sheet clusters, containing cytoplasmic mucin and basally located nuclei (Papanicolaou, ×20). (**b**) Intestinal subtype with sever atypia. High columnar cells having nuclear crowding, nuclear stratification, and hyperchromatism are observed (Papanicolaou, ×40). (**c**) Pancreatobiliary subtype with sever atypia. Neoplastic cells are arranged in large and irregular dendritic cluster, with round to oval nuclei and hyperchromatism (Papanicolaou, ×40). (**d**) Oncocytic subtype with severe atypia. Neoplastic cells having low nuclear-cytoplasmic ratio, granular cytoplasm, and hyperchromatism with large nucleolus are observed (Papanicolaou, ×100)

Other molecular assessments using pancreatic juice such as mRNAs expressions of human telomerase reverse transcriptase (hTERT) (Ohuchida et al. 2006a), sonic hedgehog (SHH) (Ohuchida et al. 2006b), S100P (Ohuchida et al. 2006c), S100A11 (Ohuchida et al. 2006d), S100A6 (Ohuchida et al. 2006e), and Twist (Ohuchida et al. 2006f), and aberrant methylations of tissue factor pathway inhibitor 2 (TFPI-2) (Jiang et al. 2006) and secreted apoptosis-related protein 2 (SARP2) (Watanabe et al. 2006) have been also attempted to improve the diagnostic ability of malignant IPMNs. Although those markers are sometimes useful to differentiate PDACs from IPMNs, or pancreatic neoplasms including PDACs and IPMNs from chronic pancreatitis, they could not distinguish malignant IPMNs from benign IPMNs.

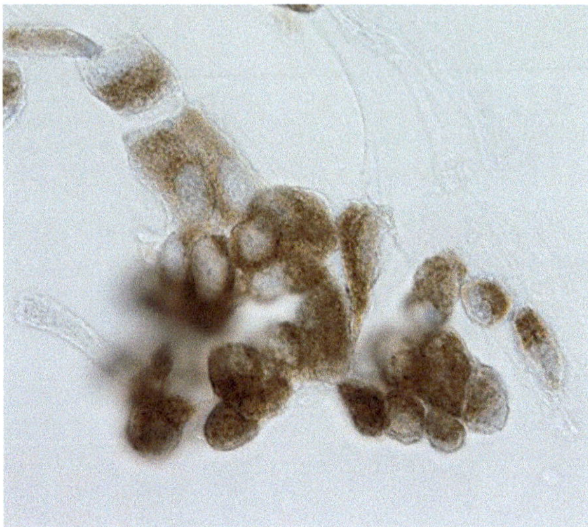

Fig. 8.4 MUC2-positive neoplastic cells in the pancreatic juice sample. Immunohistochemistry using preoperative pancreatic juice sample shows neoplasmic cells having positive staining for MUC2 (x 40). The pathological diagnosis of the resected specimen revealed intestinal subtype of IPMN (intermediate-grade dysplasia)

8.3 Intraoperative Assessment of Pancreatic Juice

IPMNs sometimes have skip lesions or concomitant PDACs which are difficult to be detected by regular imaging modalities including CT, MRI, and EUS. In these cases, intraoperative pancreatic juice cytology is useful to diagnose the presence of the unexpected lesions. Eguchi et al. (2006) used intraoperative frozen sectioning histology of cut margin and pancreatic juice cytology after secretin administration and found that 18 of 43 patients (42 %) including five with negative surgical margin but positive cytology required additional pancreatic resection during pancreatectomy for IPMNs. Our group (Mori et al. 2010) also showed the usefulness of intraoperative irrigation cytology during pancreatectomy for IPMNs to detect multifocal concomitant PDACs which were not diagnosed by preoperative imaging modalities (Fig. 8.5).

Acknowledgement The authors especially thank Dr. Shinichi Aishima and Dr. Yoshinao Oda (Department of Anatomic Pathology, Graduate School of Medical Sciences, Kyushu University) for their supports of cytological assessment of pancreatic juice and preparing the figures (Figs. 8.2c, 8.3, and 8.4) in this chapter.

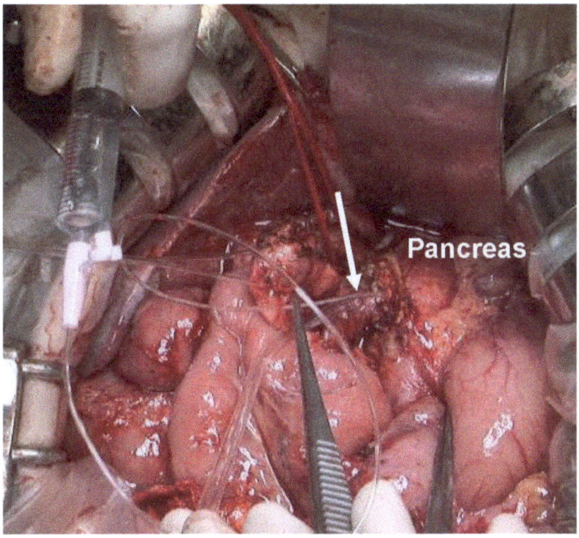

Fig. 8.5 Intraoperative pancreatic juice cytology. During pancreatoduodenectomy for IPMN in the pancreas head, the pancreas is divided at the level of portal vein, and then a 4Fr polyvinyl tube (*arrow*) is inserted into the pancreatic duct in the remnant pancreas (*distal pancreas*), and fluid for cytology is obtained by gentle irrigation of 1–2 mL of saline through a tube with a syringe

References

Ahmed K, Sussman JJ, Wang J, et al. A case of EUS-guided FNA-related pancreatic cancer metastasis to the stomach. Gastrointest Endosc. 2011;74:231–3.

Chong A, Venugopal K, Segarajasingam D, et al. Tumor seeding after EUS-guided FNA of the pancreatic tail neoplasia. Gastrointest Endosc. 2011;74:933–5.

Eguchi H, Ishikawa O, Ohigashi H, et al. Role of intraoperative cytology combined with histology in detecting continuous and skip type intraductal cancer existence for intraductal papillary mucinous carcinoma of the pancreas. Cancer. 2006;107:2567–75.

Furukawa T, Klöppel G, Adsay V, et al. Classification of types of intraductal papillary-mucinous neoplasm of the pancreas: a consensus study. Virchows Arch. 2005;447:794–9.

Furukawa T, Hatori T, Fujita I, et al. Prognostic relevance of morphological types of intraductal papillary mucinous neoplasms of the pancreas. Gut. 2011;60:509–16.

Hibi Y, Fukushima N, Tsuchida A, et al. Pancreatic juice cytology and subclassification of intraductal papillary mucinous neoplasms of the pancreas. Pancreas. 2007;34:197–204.

Hirono S, Tani M, Kawai M, et al. Treatment strategy for intraductal papillary mucinous neoplasm of the pancreas based on malignant predictive factors. Arch Surg. 2009;144:345–9.

Hirono S, Tani M, Kawai M, et al. The carcinoembryonic antigen level in pancreatic juice and mural nodule size are predictors of malignancy of branch duct type intraductal papillary mucinous neoplasms of the pancreas. Ann Surg. 2012;255:517–22.

Inoue H, Tsuchida A, Kawasaki Y, et al. Preoperative diagnosis of intraductal papillary-mucinous tumors of the pancreas with attention to telomerase activity. Cancer. 2001;91:35–41.

Jiang P, Watanabe H, Okada G, et al. Diagnostic utility of aberrant methylation of tissue factor pathway inhibitor 2 in pure pancreatic juice for pancreatic carcinoma. Cancer Sci. 2006;97: 1267–73.

Judah JR, Draganov PV. Intraductal biliary and pancreatic endoscopy: an expanding scope of possibility. World J Gastroenterol. 2008;14:3129–36.

Watanabe H, Okada G, Ohtsubo K, et al. Aberrant methylation of secreted apoptosis-related protein 2 (SARP2) in pure pancreatic juice in diagnosis of pancreatic neoplasms. Pancreas. 2006;32:382–9.

Kaino M, Kondoh S, Okita S, et al. Detection of K-ras and p53 gene mutations in pancreatic juice for the diagnosis of intraductal papillary mucinous tumors. Pancreas. 1999;18:294–9.

Kanda M, Knight S, Topazian M, et al. Mutant GNAS detected in duodenal collections of secretin-stimulated pancreatic juice indicates the presence or emergence of pancreatic cysts. Gut. 2013; 62:1024–33.

Katanuma A, Maguchi H, Hashigo S, et al. Tumor seeding after endoscopic ultrasound-guided fine-needle aspiration of cancer in the body of the pancreas. Endoscopy. 2012;44:E160–161.

Kondo H, Sugano K, Fukayama N, et al. Detection of K-ras gene mutations at codon 12 in the pancreatic juice of patients with intraductal papillary mucinous tumors of the pancreas. Cancer. 1997;79:900–5.

Kucera S, Centeno BA, Springett G, et al. Cyst fluid carcinoembryonic antigen level is not predictive of invasive cancer in patients with intraductal papillary mucinous neoplasm of the pancreas. J Periodontol. 2012;13:409–13.

Marie F, Voitot H, Aubert A, et al. Intraductal papillary mucinous neoplasms of the pancreas: performance of pancreatic fluid analysis for positive diagnosis and the prediction of malignancy. Am J Gastroenterol. 2008;103:2871–7.

Mino-Kenudson M, Fernández-del Castillo C, Baba Y, et al. Prognosis of invasive intraductal papillary mucinous neoplasm depends on histological and precursor epithelial subtypes. Gut. 2011;60:1712–20.

Mizuno O, Kawamoto H, Yamamoto N, et al. Single-pattern convergence of K-ras mutation correlates with surgical indication of intraductal papillary mucinous neoplasms. Pancreas. 2010;39:617–21.

Mori Y, Ohtsuka T, Tsutsumi K, et al. Multifocal pancreatic ductal adenocarcinomas concomitant with intraductal papillary mucinous neoplasms of the pancreas detected by intraoperative pancreatic juice cytology. A case report. J Periodontol. 2010;11:389–92.

Mori Y, Ohtsuka T, Kono H, et al. A minimally invasive and simple screening test for detection of pancreatic ductal adenocarcinoma using biomarkers in duodenal juice. Pancreas. 2013;42: 187–92.

Ohtsuka T, Ideno N, Aso T, et al. Role of endoscopic retrograde pancreatography to detect early pancreatic ductal carcinoma concomitant with intraductal papillary mucinous neoplasm of the pancreas. J Hepatobiliary Pancreat Sci. 2013;20:356–61.

Ohuchida K, Mizumoto K, Yamada D, et al. Quantitative analysis of human telomerase reverse transcriptase in pancreatic cancer. Clin Cancer Res. 2006a;12:2066–9.

Ohuchida K, Mizumoto K, Fujita H, et al. Sonic hedgehog is an early development marker of intraductal papillary mucinous neoplasms: clinical implications of mRNA levels in pancreatic juice. J Pathol. 2006b;210:42–8.

Ohuchida K, Mizumoto K, Egami T, et al. S100P is an early developmental marker of pancreatic carcinogenesis. Clin Cancer Res. 2006c;12:5411–6.

Ohuchida K, Mizumoto K, Ohhashi S, et al. S100A11, a putative tumor suppressor gene, is overexpressed in pancreatic carcinogenesis. Clin Cancer Res. 2006d;12:5417–22.

Ohuchida K, Mizumoto K, Yu J, et al. S100A6 is increased in a stepwise manner during pancreatic carcinogenesis: clinical value of expression analysis in 98 pancreatic juice samples. Cancer Epidemiol Biomarkers Prevent. 2006e;16(649):654.

Ohuchida K, Mizumoto K, Ohhashi S, et al. Twist, a novel oncogene, is upregulated in pancreatic cancer: clinical implication of Twist expression in pancreatic juice. Int J Cancer. 2006f;120:1634–40.

Paquin SC, Gariépy G, Lepanto L, et al. A first report of tumor seeding because of EUS-guided FNA of a pancreatic adenocarcinoma. Gastrointest Endosc. 2005;61:610–1.

Poultsides GA, Reddy S, Cameron JL, et al. Histopathologic basis for the favorable survival after resection of intraductal papillary mucinous neoplasm-associated invasive adenocarcinoma of the pancreas. Ann Surg. 2010;251:470–6.

Sadakari Y, Ohuchida K, Nakata K, et al. Invasive carcinoma derived from non-intestinal type intraductal papillary mucinous neoplasm of the pancreas has a poorer prognosis than that derived from intestinal type. Surgery. 2010;147:812–7.

Salla C, Chatzipantelis P, Konstantinou P, et al. Endoscopic ultrasound-guided fine-needle aspiration cytology in the diagnosis of intraductal papillary mucinous neoplasms of the pancreas. A study of 8 cases. J Periodontol. 2007;8:715–24.

Shimamoto T, Tani M, Kawai M, et al. MUC1 is a useful molecular marker for malignant intraductal papillary mucinous neoplasms in pancreatic juice obtained from endoscopic retrograde pancreatography. Pancreas. 2010;39:879–83.

Sohn TA, Yeo CJ, Cameron JL, et al. Intraductal papillary mucinous neoplasms of the pancreas. An updated experience. Ann Surg. 2004;239:788–99.

Tanaka M, Yokohata K, Konomi H, et al. Segmental balloon cytology for preoperative localization of in situ pancreatic cancer. Gastrointest Endosc. 1997;46:447–9.

Tanaka M, Fernández-del Castillo C, Adsay V, et al. International consensus guidelines 2012 for the management of IPMN and MCN of the pancreas. Pancreatology. 2012;12:183–97.

Yamaguchi K, Nakamura M, Shirahane K, et al. Pancreatic juice cytology in IPMN of the pancreas. Pancreatology. 2005a;5:416–21.

Yamaguchi T, Shirai Y, Ishihara T, et al. Pancreatic juice cytology in the diagnosis of intraductal papillary mucinous neoplasm of the pancreas: significance of sampling by peroral pancreatoscopy. Cancer. 2005b;104:2830–6.

Yopp AC, Katabi N, Janakos M, et al. Invasive carcinoma arising in intraductal papillary mucinous neoplasms of the pancreas. A match control study with conventional pancreatic ductal adenocarcinoma. Ann Surg. 2011;253:968–74.

Part III
Development of Malignancy

Chapter 9
Development of Pancreatic Carcinoma in IPMN Patients

Masao Tanaka

Abstract Patients with IPMN may synchronously or metachronously develop pancreatic ductal adenocarcinoma (PDAC) which is distinct from the IPMN. The idea of concomitant carcinoma emerged from an experience of a carcinoma in situ incidentally diagnosed by preoperative pancreatic juice cytology in a patient with a benign small branch duct (BD)-IPMN. Since then, many retrospective and prospective analyses reported the frequency of 1.9–9.2 % in various series of IPMN. The yearly incidence of concomitant PDAC has been reported to be 0.41–1.1 %. Patients at the age of >70 years and with a smaller size of BD-IPMNs and main pancreatic duct are more susceptible to the development of PDAC. The topological relationship and histological transition have been proposed for differentiation of distinct PDAC from invasive IPMN, but distinction is sometimes difficult. PDACs may frequently arise in patients with benign gastric-type IPMN in the absence of *GNAS* mutations, and so *GNAS* mutations might be useful in this context. Both of concomitant PDAC and invasive IPMN may be characterized by more favorable biological behaviors or be diagnosed earlier than ordinary PDAC. Worsening diabetes and elevation of CA 19-9 have been suggested to predict the presence of concomitant PDAC, but more sensitive markers are needed. The pancreas after resection of IPMN or concomitant PDAC is still at risk of metachronous development of PDAC. The presence of IPMN in the pancreas seems to pose the entire organ at increased risk for developing carcinoma, and then surveillance of the entire pancreas is needed to detect distinct PDAC.

Keywords Branch duct type • Concomitant pancreatic ductal adenocarcinoma • Intraductal papillary mucinous neoplasm • Malignant transformation • Pancreatic cancer

---

M. Tanaka (✉)
Department of Surgery and Oncology, Graduate School of Medical Sciences, Kyushu University, Fukuoka, Japan
e-mail: masaotan@med.kyushu-u.ac.jp

M. Tanaka (ed.), *Intraductal Papillary Mucinous Neoplasm of the Pancreas*,
DOI 10.1007/978-4-431-54472-2_9,

9.1 History

Patients with IPMN develop pancreatic carcinoma in two ways. One is well-known malignant transformation of IPMN per se and the other is the development of distinct pancreatic ductal adenocarcinoma (PDAC) in the pancreas harboring IPMN. The former is addressed in Chaps. 2 and 3. This chapter describes the features of distinct PDAC which develops in the pancreas having IPMN.

Tanaka et al. (1997) reported a patient with a branch duct (BD)-IPMN who was diagnosed as having a carcinoma in situ (CIS) by preoperative ERCP pancreatic juice cytology. This was the first case report of concomitant PDAC in a patient with a BD-IPMN. They found a CIS in a branch of the pancreatic duct near but distinct from the small benign BD-IPMN in a specimen of distal pancreatectomy (Fig. 9.1). Localization of the origin of the positive cytology was performed by repeated cytological examinations after advancing a balloon catheter into the tail portion.

Yamaguchi et al. (1997) described the significance of IPMNs as a sentinel to detect a CIS of PDAC. Five years later, they further reported the association of concomitant PDAC in seven patients with BD-IPMNs (Yamaguchi et al. 2002). Of a total of 146 patients with pancreatectomy in their series, 69 patients had IPMN alone, 70 had PDAC alone, and the other seven had both of IPMN and PDAC. The seven patients (all male) with PDAC concomitant with IPMN corresponded to 9.2 % of 76 patients with IPMN and 9.1 % of 77 patients with PDAC. IPMNs are of branch duct type in all the seven patients with a mean diameter of 3.0 cm. They are all benign adenomas with mild dysplasia. PDAC occurred synchronously with IPMN in five patients, metachronously (4 years after IPMN) in one, and synchronously with IPMN and metachronously with IPMN and PDAC (7 years after IPMN) in the other. PDACs in two of these seven patients were CIS, one minimally invasive carcinoma and the remaining four invasive carcinoma. In four of these patients,

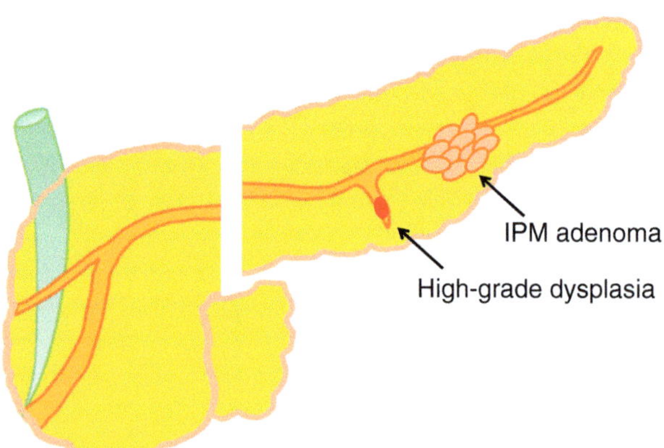

Fig. 9.1 Schematic presentation of a carcinoma in situ found by preoperative pancreatic juice cytology in a 59-year-old man with a BD-IPMN. There was a tiny area of high-grade dysplasia in a branch of the pancreatic duct near the IPMN, which proved to be low-grade dysplasia

Table 9.1 Frequency of pancreatic ductal adenocarcinoma (PDAC) in patients with branch duct IPMN

Authors (year)	Number of patients	Number of PDAC	Follow-up	Frequency (%)
Yamaguchi et al. (2002)	76	7	Retrospective analysis	9.2
Tada et al. (2006)	80	2	Retrospective analysis	2.5
Uehara et al. (2008)	60	5	Median, 87 months	8.0
Ingkakul et al. (2010)	236	22	Retrospective analysis	9.3
Tanno et al. (2010a)	168	9	Retrospective analysis	5.4
Tanno et al. (2010b)	89	4	Median, 64 months	4.5
Ikeuchi et al. (2010)	145	5	Retrospective analysis	3.5
Kanno et al. (2010)	159	7	Retrospective analysis	4.4
Sawai et al. (2010)	103	2	Retrospective analysis	1.9
Yamaguchi et al. (2011)	765	31	Retrospective analysis	4.1
Ohtsuka et al. (2012)	172	6	Retrospective analysis of patients after resection	3.5

the presence of IPMN led to the diagnosis of PDAC. Stage of the seven PDACs concomitant with IPMN was significantly earlier and the survival was better than that of the other 70 PDACs.

Since then, there have been many publications reporting the association of PDAC and IPMN (Table 9.1). The authors who first reported this phenomenon later investigated clinicopathological data of their consecutive series of 236 patients with IPMN treated by surgical resection or on follow-up to identify predictors of the presence of PDAC (Ingkakul et al. 2010). Concomitant PDAC was detected synchronously or metachronously in 22 patients (9.3 %) with BD-IPMNs (Fig. 9.2). Multivariate analysis revealed two significant factors predictive of the presence of PDAC, including worsening diabetes mellitus ($P \leq 0.001$) and an abnormal serum carbohydrate antigen (CA) 19-9 level ($P \leq 0.024$). Ikeuchi et al. (2010) reviewed the records of 145 patients with BD-IPMN observed for the mean period of 55.9±45.3 months. The frequency of extrapancreatic cancers was 29.0 % (gastric, colon, breast, 25.5 %, 15.7 %, 13.7 %, respectively). The frequency of PDAC was 9.8 %. The cause of death was extrapancreatic carcinoma in 40 %, PDAC in 25 %, IPMN per se in 20 %, and benign disease in 15 %. In another retrospective study of 103 patients with BD-IPMN conservatively followed up for ≥2 years (median 59 months) by endoscopic ultrasonography (EUS) revealed that two patients (1.9 %) developed PDAC, while four IPMNs (3.8 %) progressed into IPMC (Sawai et al. 2010). The Japan Pancreas Society (JPS) conducted a large-scale retrospective study to define the clinicopathological features of IPMC and PDAC concomitant with IPMN (Yamaguchi et al. 2011). Of 765 patients with resected IPMN, 122 patients were diagnosed as having IPMC and 31 patients (4.1 %) PDAC concomitant with IPMN. By comparison of the clinicopathological data of these patients with that of 7,605 patients with PDAC registered in the JPS pancreatic cancer registry, IPMC and PDAC concomitant with IPMN were significantly smaller, less invasive, and less extensive than ordinary PDAC. The median survival of patients with the

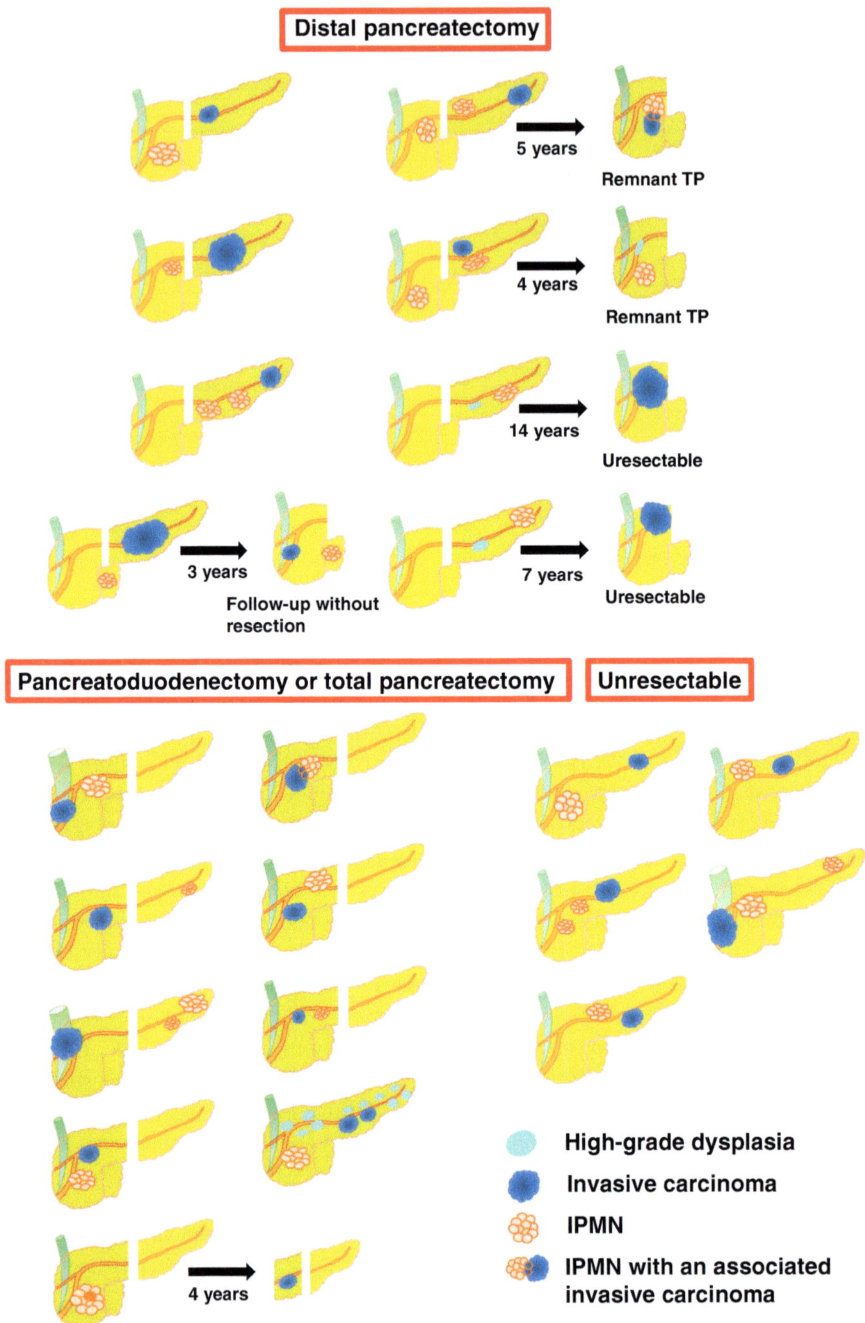

Fig. 9.2 Schematic presentation of 22 PDACs synchronously or metachronously occurring in the pancreas which harbors BD-IPMNs

former two conditions was significantly longer than for those with ordinary PDAC when compared overall or even when limited to TS2 (2.0 cm < tumor size ≤ 4.0 cm) or TS3 (4.0 cm < tumor size ≤ 6.0 cm) cases, suggesting that both of PDAC concomitant with IPMN and IPMC may have more favorable biological behaviors or be diagnosed earlier than ordinary PDAC.

Thus, in all probability, the presence of IPMN in the pancreas seems to pose the entire organ at increased risk for developing carcinoma, and surveillance of the entire pancreas is needed to detect an invasive carcinoma arising in a distinct area of the pancreas (Tada et al. 2006; Uehara et al. 2008; Ingkakul et al. 2010; Tanno et al. 2010a, b; Ikeuchi et al. 2010; Sawai et al. 2010; Yamaguchi et al. 2011; Ohtsuka et al. 2012).

9.2 The Incidence of Distinct PDAC in IPMN Patients

The incidence of PDAC development in patients with IPMNs has been estimated in a few prospective and several retrospective cohort studies. In one prospective study reported by Tada et al. (2006), 197 patients with cystic lesions including 80 IPMNs and 117 with "non-IPMN cysts" were surveyed twice a year for 3.8 years on average. Distinct PDAC developed in five patients (2.5 %, 0.68 % per year) while two IPMNs grew up to carcinoma (IPMC). Three of the five distinct PDACs developed in those with "non-IPMN cysts." Taken these PDACs and IPMCs altogether, a standardized incidence ratio (SIR) was 22.5 (95 % confidence interval, 11.0–45.3) as compared with the expected incidence calculated on the basis of age- and gender-matched mortality of pancreatic cancer in the general Japanese population. In another prospective study, 60 patients with BD-IPMN <10 mm on images and a negative cytology of the pancreatic juice were followed up mainly by ultrasonography (US) and additionally by EUS, computed tomography (CT), magnetic resonance cholangiopancreatography (MRCP), or endoscopic retrograde cholangiopancreatography (ERCP) with cytological examination of the pancreatic juice for 87 months on average (Uehara et al. 2008). PDAC distinct from IPMN developed in five patients (8 %), thus the 5-year rate of development of PDAC 6.9 % (95 % confidence interval [CI] 0.4–13.4 %), incidence of PDAC 1.1 % (95 % CI 0.1–2.2 %) per year, and SIR of PDAC 26 (95 % CI 3–48). Patients at the age of >70 years were more susceptible to the development of PDAC than those under 69. Importantly, 4 out of the 5 PDACs found during the follow-up were resectable. On the other hand, IPMNs showed malignant transformation only in 2 of 60 (3 %) BD-IPMNs. Tanno et al. (2010a) surveyed 89 patients with BD-IPMN for more than 2 years (median 64 months; range 25–158 months). PDAC developed in four patients (7.2 per 1,000 patient-years), thus the SIR in comparison with the vital statistics compiled by the Ministry of Health, Labor, and Welfare of Japan 15.8 (95 % CI, 4.3–40.4 %; P=0.00014). The incidence of PDAC was significantly greater in patients 70 years or older (SIR 16.7; 95 % CI, 3.4–48.7; P=0.0008) and in women (SIR 22.5; 95 % CI, 2.7–81.1; $P=0.0037$). The same group found PDAC in 9 (5.4 %) of 168 patients synchronously or metachronously with BD-IPMN under surveillance. The mean age of these patients was 73.1 years (range, 66–83). Patients developing PDAC were significantly older than patients not developing PDAC ($P=0.017$). The diameters of the BD-IPMNs and main pancreatic duct were significantly smaller in patients developing PDAC than those not developing PDAC ($P=0.013$ and $P<0.001$, respectively) (Tanno et al. 2010b). The JPS large-scale retrospective analysis (Maguchi et al. 2011) showed that 62 (17.8 %) of 349 patients with BD-IPMN observed or a median follow-up period of 3.7 years exhibited disease progression. PDAC and additional BD-IPMNs developed in seven (2.0 %) and 13 (3.7 %) patients, respectively, thus the yearly incidence of distinct PDAC 0.41 %.

9.3 Differentiation of Invasive IPMN and Distinct PDAC

WHO classification of IPMN pathology mentions invasive carcinoma derived from IPMNs as invasive carcinoma associated with IPMN (Adsay et al. 2010). However, the author would like to claim that the term "associated" should be defined more clearly. As we know by the aforementioned evidences, concomitant PDAC may occur in the pancreas harboring IPMNs, and this phenomenon can also be called "associated with IPMN." The author would like to propose more clear definition of carcinoma developing in the pancreas having IPMNs, i.e., invasive carcinoma derived from IPMN (identical to IPMC) and invasive carcinoma concomitant with IPMN just as we reported previously (Yamaguchi et al. 2011).

When far advanced, it is sometimes difficult to distinguish invasive IPMN (IPMC) and PDAC concomitant with IPMN. Yamaguchi et al. (2011) analyzed clinicopathological features of 765 resected IPMNs, 122 of which were diagnosed as having PDAC derived from IPMN and 31 with PDAC concomitant with IPMN. Additional 30 patients also had PDAC and IPMN, but the topological relationship and histological transition did not allow their pathologists performing central review of the histological slides to judge if the carcinoma was derived or separate from IPMN. Since there have been no other reports in regard with differentiation of PDAC derived from IPMN and distinct PDAC concomitant with IPMN, this is the current strategy and limitation of differentiation of these two types of pancreatic carcinoma. Some molecular and/or genetic analyses may be expected to contribute to more clear differentiation in the future.

9.4 Characteristics of Distinct PDAC Concomitant with IPMN

Regarding clinicopathological features of PDAC concomitant with IPMN, Yamaguchi et al. (2011) compared 122 invasive carcinomas derived from IPMN and 31 PDACs concomitant with IPMN with 7,605 patients with ordinary PDAC in the aforementioned study by the JPS. They demonstrated that both of PDACs derived from IPMN and concomitant with IPMN were significantly smaller, less invasive, and less extensive than ordinary PDACs. The median survival of patients with these two conditions was significantly longer than of those with ordinary PDAC when compared overall or even when limited to TS2 (2.0 cm < tumor size ≤ 4.0 cm) or TS3 (4.0 cm < tumor size ≤ 6.0 cm). Thus, PDAC concomitant with IPMN and PDAC derived from IPMN may be characterized by more favorable biological behaviors or be diagnosed earlier than ordinary PDAC.

There is one report analyzing imaging characteristics of IPMNs of the pancreas which develops concomitant PDAC (Tanno et al. 2010b). BD-IPMNs in patients developing distinct PDAC were characterized by the significantly smaller size of the cyst and main pancreatic duct than in patients not developing PDAC. Whether the patients with PDACs concomitant with IPMN are more likely to have multicentric carcinogenesis or not has not been determined yet, although there have been anecdotal reports of multifocal PDACs and IPMNs (Yamaguchi et al. 2005; Mori et al. 2010).

Since the vast majority of PDACs concomitant with IPMN have been reported from Japan, one may argue that there may be racial predisposition to Japanese patients. However, the same phenomenon has begun to be noticed in Western countries as well. Jarry et al. (2010) reported a patient who was diagnosed as having a symptomatic IPMN in the uncinate process and a concurrent stenosis of the neck portion of the main pancreatic duct which resulted in distal dilation. During a Whipple procedure, a concomitant adenocarcinoma was diagnosed 2 cm from the primary IPMN, causing the stenosis. Just like us, they also suggested the possibility that IPMN may be a "red flag" enabling earlier diagnosis of a concurrent PDAC arising in another area of the pancreas. Although the viewpoint was reverse, Macari et al. (2010) pointed out that IPMN occurred with increased frequency in patients with PDAC as opposed to those without PDAC. They compared the frequency of IPMN on images of 68 patients who underwent pancreatectomy for PDAC and 183 different adult patients undergoing magnetic resonance imaging (MRI) for renal mass. Five of 68 (7.3 %) patients who underwent pancreatic resection for PDAC had IPMN at a site distant from the PDAC, whereas only two of the other 183 (1.1 %) patients undergoing MRI for renal cancer had imaging evidence of IPMN. The prevalence of IPMN was significantly different ($P = 0.017$) between patients with and without PDAC, and the odds ratio for IPMN as a predictor of PDAC was estimated as 7.18.

9.5 Detection of Concomitant PDAC in Patients with IPMN

Ingkakul et al. (2010) retrospectively reviewed the clinicopathological data of 236 patients with IPMN to determine the factors predicting the presence of concomitant PDAC. When clinicopathological variables were compared between 22 IPMN patients with concomitant PDAC (9.3 %) and those without concomitant PDAC, all IPMNs concomitant with PDAC were of benign branch duct type and the histological grades of 12 resected IPMNs were low-grade ($n=8$) or intermediate-grade dysplasia ($n=4$). Multivariate analysis revealed that worsening diabetes mellitus ($P<0.001$) and an abnormal serum CA 19-9 level ($P=0.024$) were the significant predictive factors for the presence of PDAC in IPMN.

In a surveillance of BD-IPMN, how often and by what method we should examine our patients are the current issues remaining to be solved as soon as possible. A usual approach undertaken at present is blood tests for CA 19-9 and carcinoembryonic antigen (CEA) and imagings (CT, MRI/MRCP, with or without EUS) twice a year (Tada et al. 2006). However, whether this approach is appropriate and sufficient has not been determined yet. If not, what factors mandate closer intervals of surveillance must also be clarified. A family history of IPMN and/or PDAC, the growth rate of BD-IPMNs, and multiplicity of the IPMNs may be candidate factors, and there may be some other factors to be evaluated. With regard to family history of PDAC, one study reported that characteristics of surgically resected IPMNs were not different between 45 patients (13.9 %) with and 279 without a family history of PDAC (Nehra et al. 2012). Most importantly, the incidence of invasive IPMN was not different between the two groups. However, there have been very few studies to address the difference in the incidence of concomitant PDAC in patients with IPMN with and without the family history of PDAC. The growth rate of BD-IPMN has been suggested to predict the malignant change of IPMN per se (Rautou et al. 2008; Kang et al. 2011), but whether a rapidly enlarging IPMN is more likely to be associated with distinct PDAC remains unknown.

When resection is performed for an IPMN or a distinct PDAC in a patient with IPMNs, intraoperative pancreatic juice cytology should always be performed in order to confirm the absence of carcinoma in the pancreas to be left in place after planned resection. Eguchi et al. (2006) emphasized the importance of precise evaluation of intraductal cancer extension and skip lesions when resecting IPMN. Using intraoperative frozen section histology and pancreatic juice cytology, 18 out of 43 patients (42 %) required additional resection of the pancreas. Logistic regression analysis revealed that patients with a dilated main pancreatic duct, or those with cancerous lesions in the main tumors, were at high risk for positive histology and/or cytology. Mori et al. (2010) also reported a patient with multifocal PDACs concomitant with IPMN detected by intraoperative pancreatic juice cytology. Later, the same authors evaluated the technique of intraoperative irrigation cytology of the remnant pancreas to detect distinct PDAC during pancreatectomy in patients with IPMN (Mori et al. 2013). Of 48 patients who underwent irrigation cytology of the remnant pancreas during pancreatectomy, 13 patients had suspicious or positive results at the first attempt. Eight of these subsequently had negative results at the second or third attempt, while five patients (10 %) continued to show positive results, necessitating additional resection. All five patients had a distinct PDAC in the additionally resected specimen, none of which were detected by preoperative imaging studies. Noteworthy is the fact that four of these five PDACs were stage 0 or 1.

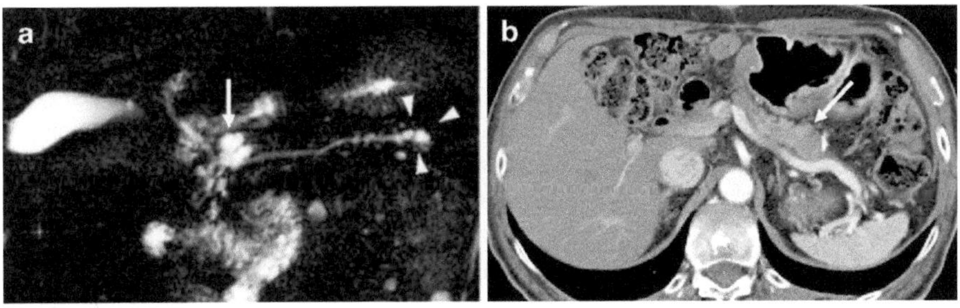

Fig. 9.3 Metachronous development of a PDAC in the remnant pancreas after resection of IPMNs in a 72-year-old man. Based on pancreatic juice cytology positive for Class IV, pylorus-preserving pancreatoduodenectomy was performed for a 15-mm BD-IPMN (**a**, *arrow*) of low-grade dysplasia as well as pancreatic tail resection for a 12-mm BD-IPMN (**a**, *arrowheads*) of high-grade dysplasia. During postoperative surveillance twice a year, a solid mass with delayed enhancement was detected near the margin of the tail of the pancreas 15 months later (**b**, *arrow*). Histological examination after remnant pancreatectomy revealed a well to moderately differentiated adenocarcinoma. The margin of the previous pancreatic tail resection was free from IPMN and the metachronous carcinoma did not reach the stump of the pancreatic tail

9.6 Development of PDAC after Resection of IPMN

The pancreas remaining after resection of IPMN with negative resection margins or after resection of PDAC concomitant with IPMN is still at risk of metachronous development of PDAC as well as IPMN. Miller et al. (2011) surveyed 153 patients who underwent resection for IPMN with negative margins. During a mean period of 73 months, 31 of the 153 (20 %) patients developed a new IPMN and three of them proved to be invasive cancer. Ohtsuka et al. (2012) reviewed 172 patients who underwent resection of IPMNs with a mean postoperative follow-up of 64 months. Ten metachronous IPMNs developed in the remnant pancreas after a mean time of 23 postoperative months, and two with main duct IPMNs (both were CIS) required remnant pancreatectomy. On the other hand, six distinct PDACs developed in the remnant pancreas of these 172 patients after a mean time of 84 postoperative months (range, 12–150 months). Four of them were found to have a tumor with a size <2 cm (Fig. 9.3), whereas the remaining two PDACs were found to be unresectable more than 10 years after resection of IPMNs. Intense long-term surveillance is necessary for early detection of metachronous occurrence of distinct PDACs as well as malignant IPMNs after resection of IPMNs.

9.7 Molecular Aspects of Development of PDAC in IPMN Patients

KRAS mutations are frequently detected in both PDACs and IPMNs (Tada et al. 1991; Mizuno et al. 2010). Several molecular studies showed heterogeneity within the pancreas with IPMN, demonstrating multiple subclones evidenced by the presence of several different *KRAS* mutations (Wu et al. 2011a, b; Lubezky et al. 2011; Matthaei et al. 2012). However, few studies have investigated molecular alterations within IPMNs and synchronously or metachronously occurring distinct PDACs. *KRAS* mutations are present in 30–80 % of IPMNs, and *GNAS* mutations of codon 201, unique to IPMNs, have been detected in more than 60 % of IPMNs (Furukawa et al. 2011; Wu et al. 2011a, b). Wu et al. (2011a, b) carefully microdissected neoplastic cells of IPMN and invasive carcinoma derived from IPMN in eight patients and purified DNA. In seven of the eight patients (88 %), identical *GNAS* mutation was found in the neoplastic cells of the IPMN and invasive carcinoma derived from the IPMN. *KRAS* mutation of the PDAC was consistent with that of the associated IPMN in these patients. Although the *KRAS* mutations are found commonly in both PDACs derived from IPMN and PDACs not associated with IPMN, there was a marked difference between the prevalence of *GNAS* mutations in PDACs associated with IPMN (7 of 8) and that in PDACs unassociated with IPMN (0 of 116; $P<0.001$). In the eighth patient, however, the *KRAS* and *GNAS* mutations identified in the neoplastic cells of the IPMN were not found in the PDAC, suggesting that this invasive cancer arose from a separate precursor lesion. Lubezky et al. (2011) found concordant *KRAS* mutations in IPMNs and carcinoma derived from the IPMNs in 9 of 14 patients (64 %). Ideno et al. (2013) reviewed clinicopathological data of 179 resected IPMNs and 180 resected PDACs without IPMNs. Twenty-six synchronous or metachronous PDACs were identified in 20 patients (11.2 %) with IPMNs in their series. Occurrence of concomitant PDACs was more frequently observed in gastric-type IPMNs (18/110, 16.4 %) compared with intestinal (1/49, 2.0 %), pancreatobiliary (1/17, 5.9 %), or oncocytic type (0/3, 0 %) ($P=0.047$). The mucin-staining patterns were similar to those of invasive tubular adenocarcinoma arising from gastric-type IPMNs, being frequently positive for MUC1, MUC5AC, and MUC6 expression but negative for MUC2 and CDX2. Mutation of *GNAS* within codon 201 was not detected in PDACs and gastric-type IPMNs, while most of these exhibited *KRAS* mutations. However, the R201H *GNAS* mutation was detected in one intestinal-type IPMN with distinct PDAC. PDACs may frequently arise in the pancreas with benign gastric-type IPMN in the absence of *GNAS* mutations. All these data suggest that *GNAS* mutations might be useful to distinguish PDACs derived from IPMN (*KRAS* mutation+, *GNAS* mutation+) and PDACs concomitant with but distinct from IPMN (*KRAS* mutation+, *GNAS* mutation-) in most cases.

Matthaei et al. (2012) investigated the clonal relationships of 30 multifocal IPMNs arising in 13 patients. The majority of multifocal IPMNs were of branch duct type of gastric subtype with low or intermediate grades of dysplasia. *KRAS* mutation analysis and loss of heterozygosity (LOH) analysis on chromosomes 6*q* and 17*p* on these multiple IPMNs showed non-overlapping *KRAS* gene mutations in eight patients (62 %) and discordant LOH profiles in seven patients (54 %), thus depicting independent genetic alterations in 9 of the 13 patients (69 %).

9.8 Prevention of PDAC Concomitant with IPMN

A role for medical management of IPMNs such as chemoprevention remains an unanswered question. Although there have been clinical trials of chemoprevention conducted for a variety of malignancies, only one study examined the effect of sulindac in a series of 22 patients with BD-IPMNs (Hayashi et al. 2009). Ten of 22 patients who rejected surgical therapy despite their lesions meeting the Sendai criteria for surgical resection were assigned to the treatment group. Sulindac (150 mg twice daily) and omeprazole (20 mg once daily) were administered for 18 months, while the other 12 patients served as controls. The cyst size and height of mural nodules of BD-IPMNs monitored by MRCP or CT and EUS were significantly reduced in the treatment group, while those in the control group remained unchanged, suggesting the promise of chemoprevention of carcinoma derived from BD-IPMNs by sulindac. Immunohistochemical staining for cyclooxygenase-1 and cyclooxygenase-2 was negative in hyperplasia, adenoma, and carcinoma portions of resected specimens but was clearly positive for glutathione-S-transferase pi (GST-pi), suggesting that GST-pi is a putative target molecule for sulindac.

References

Adsay NV, Kloppel G, Fukushima N, et al. Intraductal papillary-mucinous neoplasms of the pancreas. In: Bosman FT et al., editors. World health organization classification of tumors, pathology and genetics of tumors of the digestive system. Lyon: IARC; 2010. p. 304–13.

Eguchi H, Ishikawa O, Ohigashi H, et al. Role of intraoperative cytology combined with histology in detecting continuous and skip type intraductal cancer existence for intraductal papillary mucinous carcinoma of the pancreas. Cancer. 2006;107:2567–75.

Furukawa T, Kuboki Y, Tanji E, et al. Whole-exome sequencing uncovers frequent GNAS mutations in intraductal papillary mucinous neoplasms of the pancreas. Sci Rep. 2011;1:161.

Hayashi T, Ishiwatari H, Ihara H, et al. Suppressive effect of sulindac on branch duct-intraductal papillary mucinous neoplasms. J Gastroenterol. 2009;44:964–75.

Ideno N, Ohtsuka T, Kono H et al. Intraductal papillary mucinous neoplasms of the pancreas with distinct pancreatic ductal adenocarcinomas are frequently of gastric subtype. Ann Surg. 2013; 258:141–51.

Ikeuchi N, Itoi T, Sofuni A, et al. Prognosis of cancer with branch duct type IPMN of the pancreas. World J Gastroenterol. 2010;16:1890–5.

Ingkakul T, Sadakari Y, Ienaga J, et al. Predictors of the presence of concomitant invasive ductal carcinoma in intraductal papillary mucinous neoplasm of the pancreas. Ann Surg. 2010;251:70–5.

Jarry J, Belleannee G, Rault A, et al. Can an intraductal papillary mucinous tumor be a potential indicator of concurrent adenocarcinoma of the pancreas? J Periodontol. 2010;11:55–7.

Kang MJ, Jang JY, Kim SJ, et al. Cyst growth rate predicts malignancy in patients with branch duct intraductal papillary mucinous neoplasms. Clin Gastroenterol Hepatol. 2011;9:87–93.

Kanno A, Satoh K, Hirota M, et al. Prediction of invasive carcinoma in branch type intraductal papillary mucinous neoplasms of the pancreas. J Gastroenterol. 2010;45:952–59

Lubezky N, Ben-Haim M, Marmor S, et al. High-throughput mutation profiling in intraductal papillary mucinous neoplasm (IPMN). J Gastrointest Surg. 2011;15:503–11.

Macari M, Eubig J, Robinson E, et al. Frequency of intraductal papillary mucinous neoplasm in patients with and without pancreas cancer. Pancreatology. 2010;10:734–41.

Maguchi H, Tanno S, Mizuno N, et al. Natural history of branch duct intraductal papillary mucinous neoplasms of the pancreas: a multicenter study in Japan. Pancreas. 2011;40:364–70.

Matthaei H, Norris AL, Tsiatis AC, et al. Clinicopathological characteristics and molecular analyses of multifocal intraductal papillary mucinous neoplasms of the pancreas. Ann Surg. 2012;255:326–33.

Miller JR, Meyer JE, Waters JA, et al. Outcome of the pancreatic remnant following segmental pancreatectomy for non-invasive intraductal papillary mucinous neoplasm. HPB (Oxford). 2011;13:759–66.

Mizuno O, Kawamoto H, Yamamoto N, et al. Single-pattern convergence of K-ras mutation correlates with surgical indication of intraductal papillary mucinous neoplasms. Pancreas. 2010;39:617–21.

Mori Y, Ohtsuka T, Tsutsumi K, et al. Multifocal pancreatic ductal adenocarcinomas concomitant with intraductal papillary mucinous neoplasms of the pancreas detected by intraoperative pancreatic juice cytology. A case report. J Periodontol. 2010;11:389–92.

Mori Y, Ohtsuka T, Tamura K et al. Intraoperative irrigation cytology of the remnant pancreas to detect distinct pancreatic ductal adenocarcinoma during pancreatectomy in patients having intraductal papillary mucinous neoplasm. Surgery. 2013 (in press)

Nehra D, Oyarvide VM, Mino-Kenudson M, et al. Intraductal papillary mucinous neoplasms: does a family history of pancreatic cancer matter? Pancreatology. 2012;12:358–63.

Ohtsuka T, Kono H, Tanabe R, et al. Follow-up study after resection of intraductal papillary mucinous neoplasm of the pancreas; special references to the multifocal lesions and development of ductal carcinoma in the remnant pancreas. Am J Surg. 2012;204:44–8.

Rautou PE, Levy P, Vullierme MP, et al. Morphologic changes in branch duct intraductal papillary mucinous neoplasms of the pancreas: a midterm follow-up study. Clin Gastroenterol Hepatol. 2008;6:807–14.

Sawai Y, Yamao K, Bhatia V, et al. Development of pancreatic cancers during long-term follow-up of side-branch intraductal papillary mucinous neoplasms. Endoscopy. 2010;42:1077–84.

Tada M, Omata M, Ohto M. Ras gene mutations in intraductal papillary mucinous neoplasms of the pancreas: analysis in five cases. Cancer. 1991;67:634–7.

Tada M, Kawabe T, Arizumi M, et al. Pancreatic cancer in patients with pancreatic cystic lesions: a prospective study in 197 patients. Clin Gastroenterol Hepatol. 2006;4:1265–70.

Tanaka M, Yokohata K, Konomi H, et al. Segmental balloon cytology for preoperative localization of in situ pancreatic cancer. Gastrointest Endosc. 1997;46:447–9.

Tanno S, Nakano Y, Koizumi K, et al. Pancreatic ductal adenocarcinomas in long-term follow-up patients with branch duct intraductal papillary mucinous neoplasms. Pancreas. 2010a;39:36–40.

Tanno S, Nakano Y, Sugiyama Y, et al. Incidence of synchronous and metachronous pancreatic carcinoma in 168 patients with branch duct intraductal papillary mucinous neoplasm. Pancreatology. 2010b;10:173–8.

Uehara H, Nakaizumi A, Ishikawa O, et al. Development of ductal carcinoma of the pancreas during follow-up of branch duct intraductal papillary mucinous neoplasm of the pancreas. Gut. 2008;57:1561–5.

Wu J, Matthaei H, Maitra A, et al. Recurrent GNAS mutations define an unexpected pathway for pancreatic cyst development. Sci Transl Med. 2011a;3:92ra66.

Wu J, Jiao Y, Dal Molin M, et al. Whole-exome sequencing of neoplastic cysts of the pancreas reveals recurrent mutations in components of ubiquitin-dependent pathways. Proc Natl Acad Sci USA. 2011b;108:21188–93.

Yamaguchi K, Nakamura K, Yokohata K, et al. Pancreatic cyst as a sentinel of in situ carcinoma of the pancreas. Report of two cases. Int J Pancreatol. 1997;22:227–31.

Yamaguchi K, Ohuchida J, Ohtsuka T, et al. Intraductal papillary-mucinous tumor of the pancreas concomitant with ductal carcinoma of the pancreas. Pancreatology. 2002;2:484–90.

Yamaguchi K, Konomi H, Kobayashi K, et al. Total pancreatectomy for intraductal papillary-mucinous tumor of the pancreas: reappraisal of total pancreatectomy. Hepatogastroenterology. 2005;52:1585–90.

Yamaguchi K, Kanemitsu S, Hatori T, et al. Pancreatic ductal adenocarcinoma derived from IPMN and pancreatic ductal adenocarcinoma concomitant with IPMN. Pancreas. 2011;40:571–80.

Chapter 10
Development of Extrapancreatic Malignancy

Koji Yamaguchi

Abstract Over the past two decades, multiple studies have demonstrated an increased incidence of additional malignancies in patients with intraductal papillary mucinous neoplasm (IPMN). The majority of these additional cancers occur before or concurrent with the diagnosis of IPMN. The gastrointestinal tract is most commonly involved in secondary malignancies, with benign colon polyps and colon cancer commonly seen in Western countries and gastric cancer commonly seen in Asian countries. Other extrapancreatic malignancies associated with IPMN include benign and malignant esophageal neoplasms, gastrointestinal stromal tumors, carcinoid tumors, hepatobiliary cancers, breast cancers, prostate cancers, and lung cancers. There is no clear etiology for the development of secondary malignancies in patients with IPMN. Although population-based studies have shown different results from single-institution studies regarding the exact incidence of additional primary cancers in IPMN patients, both have reached the same conclusion: there is a higher incidence of extrapancreatic malignancies in patients with IPMN than in the general population. This finding has significant clinical implications for both the initial evaluation and subsequent long-term follow-up in patients with IPMN. At present, there are no recommended screening modalities for detecting extrapancreatic malignancies; however, once the diagnosis is made, the possibility of extrapancreatic neoplasms should be considered based on the frequency of malignancy in the general population of the country or region.

Keywords Extrapancreatic malignancy • IPMN

K. Yamaguchi (✉)
Department of Surgery, School of Medicine, University of Occupational and Environmental Health, 1-1 Iseigaoka, Yahatanishi-ku, Kitakyushu 807-8555, Japan
e-mail: yamaguch@med.uoeh-u.ac.jp

DOI 10.1007/978-4-431-54472-2_10, © Springer Japan 2014

10.1 Incidence of Extrapancreatic Malignancy

The synchronous and metachronous occurrence of malignant diseases in extrapancreatic organs in patients with IPMN has an incidence of 10–45 % (Fig. 10.1) (Sugiyama and Atomi 1999; Choi et al. 2006; Eguchi et al. 2006; Lee et al. 2006; Riall et al. 2007; Ishida et al. 2008; Yoon et al. 2008; Baumgaertner et al. 2008; Oh et al. 2009; Reid-Lombardo et al. 2010; Calculli et al. 2010; Lubezky et al. 2012). Table 10.1 shows the incidence of extrapancreatic malignancies reported in the English literature. The incidence is similar around the world. In our series of 48

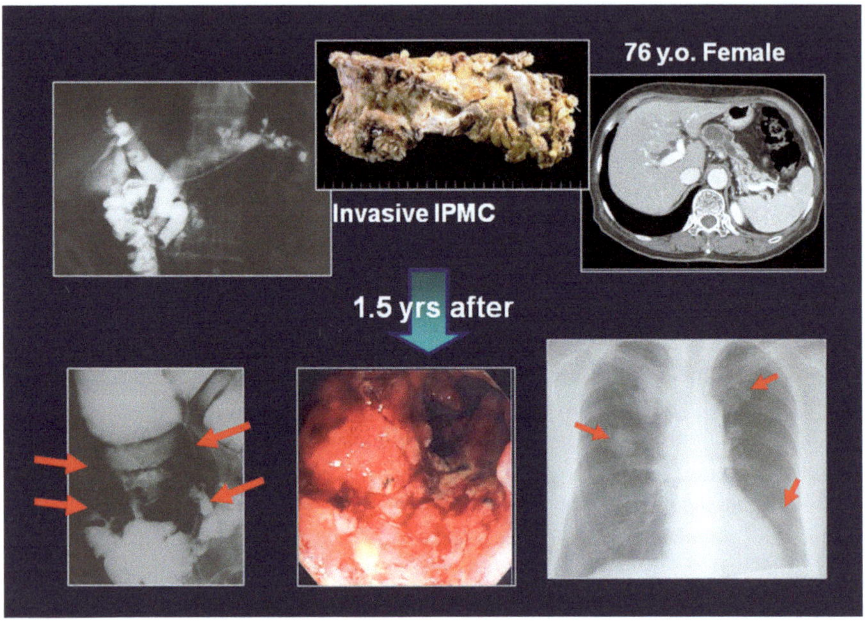

Fig. 10.1 Colon cancer 1.5 years after resection of IPMN

Table 10.1 Extrapancreatic malignancies of IPMN

Sugiyama M	1999	Japan	42	14	32 %
Choi MG	2006	Korea	61	24	39 %
Eguchi H	2006	Japan	69	31	45 %
Lee SY	2006	Korea	54	7	13 %
Riall TS	2007	USA	983	99	10.1 %
Ishida M	2008	Japan	61	15	25 %
Yoon WJ	2008	Korea	210	71	33.8 %
Baumgaertner	2008	France	178	30	16.8 %
Oh SJ	2009	Korea	37	10	27 %
Reid-Lombardo KM	2010	USA	471	183	38.9 %
Calculi L	2010	Italy	142	12	8.5 %
Lubezky	2012	Israel	82	16	19.5 %

patients with IPMN, 13 (27 %) had synchronous or metachronous extrapancreatic malignancies (Yamaguchi et al. 1999). In our recent series of 101 patients with surgically proven IPMN, 22 (22 %) had extrapancreatic malignancies. The incidence remained almost the same, even after the number of patients with IPMN increased.

Whether the true incidence of extrapancreatic malignancy is higher remains controversial. All single-institution studies were retrospective and had relatively small numbers of patients with IPMN. Based on their design, retrospective studies are limited by the fact that complete data can be missed if a history of prior cancer is not documented. In addition, follow-up data are limited if the patients go elsewhere for diagnosis and/or treatment of additional neoplasms after receiving treatment for IPMN. Moreover, it is conceivable that the patients seen at referral centers differ from and undergo different treatments than the general population. At referral centers, such as the Mayo Clinic, the number of patients treated for IPMN is high compared with that observed at non-referral centers; however, such referral centers have limitations (Reid-Lombardo et al. 2010).

Population-based studies also have inherent limitations. The correct classification of IPMN relative to other cystic pancreatic neoplasms was unclear until 1996, when the World Health Organization defined clear criteria for its diagnosis (Kloeppel et al. 1996). A US population-based study included patients from 1983 to 1991 to follow all patients for 10 years in order to determine the incidence of extrapancreatic malignancies after the diagnosis of IPMN. It is possible that many IPMNs were misclassified (Riall et al. 2007). In addition, this study included only invasive cases of IPMN since benign cases of IPMN are not registered in the SEER database. A case-controlled study concerning a large series of 178 IPMN patients who underwent resection matched with 356 controls demonstrated a higher prevalence of extrapancreatic malignancies in the IPMN patients than in the control group (Baumgaertner et al. 2008). Eguchi et al. (2006) calculated the rate of increase in the incidence of extrapancreatic malignancies in IPMN patients compared with that observed in the normal population using the Osaka Cancer Registry, one of the largest cancer databases. The O/E ratio of preoperative colorectal cancer was significantly higher in the IPMN patients (5.37; 95 % confidence interval, 2.31–10.58).

10.2 Location of Extrapancreatic Malignancies

The frequency and location of extrapancreatic malignancies differ from country to country (Table 10.2) (Eguchi et al. 2006; Yoon et al. 2008; Baumgaertner et al. 2008; Reid-Lombardo et al. 2010; Lubezky et al. 2012; Kamisawa et al. 2005). Gastrointestinal cancer is common in Asia, while skin, breast, and prostate cancers are frequent in the United States (Benarroch-Gampel and Riall 2010). These facts may indicate that extrapancreatic malignancies occur depending on the incidence of cancer in the general population in the different regions. A case-controlled study concerning a large series of 178 IPMN patients who underwent resection matched with 356 controls showed that the type of extrapancreatic malignancy was not different between the IPMN and control groups (Baumgaertner et al. 2008).

Table 10.2 Extrapancreatic malignancies of IPMN

	Japan		Korea	Israel	France	USA
	Kamisawa ($n=37$)	Eguchi ($n=32$)	Yoon ($n=77$)	Lubezky ($n=16$)	Baumgaertner ($n=30$)	Reid-Lombardo ($n=192$)
Colorectum	7	8	16	5	3	19
Stomach	12	4	29			
Lung	4	5			3	3
Bile duct	1		7			
Esophagus	4					9
Kidney		2		1		
Prostate	1	2		3		24
Urinary bladder		2			4	
Liver	2					8
Breast	2			3	9	24
Others	4	9	25	4	11	[a]105

[a]Including 35 nonmelanoma skin, 14 gynecologic, 11 hematologic, and six carcinoid

Table 10.3 The diagnosis of extrapancreatic malignancies of IPMN

	Before Dx of IPMN	Synchronous with IPMN	After Dx of IPMN
Sugiyama ($n=15$)	7	3	5
Kamisawa ($n=37$)	15	19	6
Choi ($n=18$)	4	12	2
Yoon ($n=77$)	21	51	5
Baumgaertner ($n=30$)	19	11	0
Ishida ($n=16$)	7	5	4

10.3 Timing of Diagnosis of Extrapancreatic Malignancy

Most reports describe the occurrence of malignant conditions as part of the patient's past history (Calculli et al. 2010) (Tables 10.3) (Sugiyama and Atomi 1999; Choi et al. 2006; Ishida et al. 2008; Yoon et al. 2008; Baumgaertner et al. 2008; Kamisawa et al. 2005). However, extrapancreatic malignancies can occur even after resection of IPMN. Therefore, attention should be paid to this phenomenon, even after resection of IPMN.

10.4 Relationship Between the Types of IPMN and Extrapancreatic Malignancy

The relationship between the types of IPMN and extrapancreatic malignancies is controversial. Some authors have reported that extrapancreatic malignancies occur in patients with all types of IPMN (Calculli et al. 2010), while others have reported that IPMA is closely associated with extrapancreatic malignancy (Ishida et al. 2008).

10.5 Etiology and Risk of Extrapancreatic Malignancy

Several authors have reported that patients with IPMN and extrapancreatic malignancies are older than patients with IPMN without extrapancreatic malignancies (Choi et al. 2006; Eguchi et al. 2006; Riall et al. 2007; Oh et al. 2009; Yoon et al. 2008). Female and white patients with IPMN have an increased risk of extrapancreatic malignancies (Riall et al. 2007).

Genetic studies have identified two potentially high-risk groups. Lee et al. (2006) recommended more intense screening for extrapancreatic malignancy in patients with IPMN who are positive for MUC2. In addition, patients with FAP may be at high risk for the development of IPMN. Further studies are needed to make specific recommendations, although patients with FAP already receive close surveillance. Identifying pancreatic cystic lesions in this group should raise suspicion for IPMN in the setting of identified mutations in the APC gene. In a recent study evaluating the gene expression in patients with IPMN, no differences were found in the p53, p21, Bd-2, or MUC5AC expression among IPMN patients with or without extrapancreatic malignancies (Lee et al. 2006).

Patients with IPMN may also share environmental risks for the development of extrapancreatic malignancies. Further genetic and environmental studies are needed to elucidate the etiology of IPMN.

10.6 Prognosis of Patients with IPMN and Extrapancreatic Malignancies

Among patients with IPMN, those with IPMC die from IPMC, while those with IPMA die from other benign conditions or extrapancreatic malignancies (Table 10.4) (Sugiyama and Atomi 1999; Choi et al. 2006; Eguchi et al. 2006; Ishida et al. 2008; Kamisawa et al. 2005). Therefore, extrapancreatic malignancy may be a possible prognostic factor in patients with IPMN. Among patients who develop secondary malignancies, approximately 2–15 % die from the lesions (Sugiyama and Atomi 1999; Choi et al. 2006; Eguchi et al. 2006; Kamisawa et al. 2005).

Table 10.4 Causes of death of patients with IPMN

	IPMC	Other malignancies	Other benign diseases
Sugiyama	2/42	1/42	3/42
Kamisawa	5/79	14/79	4/79
Eguchi		3/69	
Choi	3/61	3/61	1/61
Ishida	2/61	3/61	1/61

10.7 Screening for Extrapancreatic Malignancies

At present, there are no screening recommendations for detecting extrapancreatic malignancies; however, once the diagnosis is made, the possibility of extrapancreatic neoplasms should be considered based on the frequency of malignancies in the general population of the country or region. For patients in Asian countries, esophagogastric duodenography should be performed as part of the preoperative workup. Two reports recommend screening for colorectal polyps and cancer in the United States (Reid-Lombardo et al. 2010; Khan et al. 2010). Mammography for breast cancer and prostate-specific antigen testing and digital rectal examinations for prostate cancer should also be performed in the United States.

References

Baumgaertner I, Corcos O, Couvelard A, et al. Prevalence of extrapancreatic cancers in patients with histologically proven intraductal papillary mucinous neoplasms of the pancreas: a case–control study. Am J Gastroenterol. 2008;103(11):2878–82.

Benarroch-Gampel J, Riall TS. Extrapancreatic malignancies and intraductal papillary mucinous neoplasms of the pancreas. World J Gastrointest Surg. 2010;2(10):363–7.

Calculli L, Pezzilli R, Brindisi C, Morabito R, Casadei R, Zompatori M. Pancreatic and extrapancreatic lesions in patients with intraductal papillary mucinous neoplasms of the pancreas: a single-centre experience. Radiol Med. 2010;115(3):442–52.

Choi MG, Kim SW, Han SS, Jang JY, Park YH. High incidence of extrapancreatic neoplasms in patients with intraductal papillary mucinous neoplasms. Arch Surg. 2006;141(1):51–6. discussion 56.

Eguchi H, Ishikawa O, Ohigashi H, et al. Patients with pancreatic intraductal papillary mucinous neoplasms are at high risk of colorectal cancer development. Surgery. 2006;139(6):749–54.

Ishida M, Egawa S, Kawaguchi K, et al. Synchronous and metachronous extrapancreatic malignant neoplasms in patients with intraductal papillary-mucinous neoplasm of the pancreas. Pancreatology. 2008;8(6):577–82.

Kamisawa T, Tu Y, Egawa N, Nakajima H, Tsuruta K, Okamoto A. Malignancies associated with intraductal papillary mucinous neoplasm of the pancreas. World J Gastroenterol. 2005;11(36):5688–90.

Khan S, Sclabas G, Reid-Lombardo KM. Population-based epidemiology, risk factors and screening of intraductal papillary mucinous neoplasm patients. World J Gastrointest Surg. 2010;2(10):314–8.

Kloeppel GSE, Longnecker DS, Capella C, Sobin LH. World health organization international histological classification of tumours histological typing of tumours of exocrine pancreas. 2nd ed. Berlin: Springer; 1996.

Lee SY, Choi DW, Jang KT, et al. High expression of intestinal-type mucin (MUC2) in intraductal papillary mucinous neoplasms coexisting with extrapancreatic gastrointestinal cancers. Pancreas. 2006;32(2):186–9.

Lubezky N, Ben-Haim M, Lahat G, et al. Intraductal papillary mucinous neoplasm of the pancreas: associated cancers, family history, genetic predisposition? Surgery. 2012;151(1):70–5.

Oh SJ, Lee SJ, Lee HY, et al. Extrapancreatic tumors in intraductal papillary mucinous neoplasm of the pancreas. Korean J Gastroenterol. 2009;54(3):162–6.

Reid-Lombardo KM, Mathis KL, Wood CM, Harmsen WS, Sarr MG. Frequency of extrapancreatic neoplasms in intraductal papillary mucinous neoplasm of the pancreas: implications for management. Ann Surg. 2010;251(1):64–9.

Riall TS, Stager VM, Nealon WH, et al. Incidence of additional primary cancers in patients with invasive intraductal papillary mucinous neoplasms and sporadic pancreatic adenocarcinomas. J Am Coll Surg. 2007;204(5):803–13. discussion 13–4.

Sugiyama M, Atomi Y. Extrapancreatic neoplasms occur with unusual frequency in patients with intraductal papillary mucinous tumors of the pancreas. Am J Gastroenterol. 1999;94(2):470–3.

Yamaguchi K, Chijiiwa K, Shimizu S, et al. Intraductal papillary neoplasm of the pancreas: a clinical review of 13 benign and four malignant tumours. Eur J Surg. 1999;165(3):223–9.

Yoon WJ, Ryu JK, Lee JK, et al. Extrapancreatic malignancies in patients with intraductal papillary mucinous neoplasm of the pancreas: prevalence, associated factors, and comparison with patients with other pancreatic cystic neoplasms. Ann Surg Oncol. 2008;15(11):3193–8.

Chapter 11
Surveillance of Branch-Duct IPMN: Methods and Frequency

Walter G. Park and Suresh Chari

Abstract Branch-duct intraductal papillary mucinous neoplasms (BD-IPMNs) are common premalignant cystic lesions of the pancreas. Most are incidentally discovered. The prevalence of malignancy at the time of initial identification of BD-IPMNs is very low and they harbor little threat of imminent malignant transformation. Therefore, despite their premalignant nature, immediate surgical resection for all BD-IPMNs is not recommended as the morbidity and mortality of surgery far outweigh the likely benefit of cancer prevention. The possibility of missing an opportunity to surgically cure early cancer, however, is a challenge given our limited understanding of the natural history along with suboptimal diagnostic tools. Consensus criteria for surveillance of BD-IPMNs and indications for surgery have been proposed in 2006 (a.k.a. Sendai criteria) and recently revised in 2012 (a.k.a. Fukuoka criteria). While the evidence to support current recommendations is limited, the trend of available data continues to support deliberate observation for most BD-IPMNs without high-risk stigmata or worrisome features of malignancy. Newer diagnostic tools with better accuracy for diagnosing BD-IPMNs and their dysplasia status are needed to improve clinical management.

Keywords Branch duct • Intraductal papillary mucinous neoplasm • Surveillance

11.1 Introductory Remarks: Rationale for Surveillance

This chapter will discuss current algorithms for monitoring branch-duct intraductal papillary mucinous neoplasms (BD-IPMN) and indications for surgical resection. BD-IPMNs are one of the most common pancreatic cysts and the primary reason to

W.G. Park (✉)
Stanford University School of Medicine, Stanford, CA, USA
e-mail: wgpark@stanford.edu

S. Chari
Mayo Clinic, Rochester, MN, USA

M. Tanaka (ed.), *Intraductal Papillary Mucinous Neoplasm of the Pancreas*,
DOI 10.1007/978-4-431-54472-2_11, © Springer Japan 2014

follow them is for their recognized potential to transform into pancreatic cancer, the fourth leading cause of cancer death in the United States with an estimated annual incidence of 43,920 people and annual mortality of 37,390 in 2012 (Howlader et al. 2012). While premalignant pancreatic cysts including BD-IPMNs are thought to represent a minority of precursor lesions (~15 %), early diagnosis of malignancy and surgical resection leads to a significant 5-year survival benefit of 90–100 % (Adsay 2007; Chari et al. 2002).

Despite being a premalignant lesion of a lethal cancer, most BD-IPMNs are currently observed rather than removed by surgery because of two primary reasons. The first involves what is currently known about the natural history of BD-IPMNs (please refer to Chap. 3 for more detail). Although studies of the natural history are limited by follow-up and sample size, the current best estimates suggest an indolent course with infrequent malignant transformation of approximately 1 % per year (Al-Haddad et al. 2011; Khannoussi et al. 2012). The second reason involves the inability to remove them without incurring significant mortality and morbidity. Unlike a precancerous colon polyp or Barrett's esophagus, there is currently no minimally invasive means to resect a pancreatic cyst. Pancreatic surgery is associated with a perioperative mortality rate of 5 % and perioperative morbidity rate of 40 % (McPhee et al. 2007; Venkat et al. 2012).

With increasing use of high-resolution abdominal imaging modalities such as computed tomography (CT) and magnetic resonance imaging (MRI), there is increasing recognition of pancreatic cysts, including BD-IPMNs. Their management continues to be a clinical conundrum. In the United States, the best estimates of the prevalence of pancreatic cysts in the general population are that it is approximately 2.5 %, rising to about 9 % in the elderly (Laffan et al. 2008; de Jong et al. 2010). Until a novel technology evolves that can safely and adequately eradicate premalignant cysts, there will remain a clinical need to develop guidelines for monitoring BD-IPMNs. These guidelines should be evidence based to optimize patient benefit and minimize their risk.

11.2 The Ideal Surveillance Strategy

To better understand the challenges of developing surveillance strategies for BD-IPMNs, it helps to define important features of an ideal monitoring program. First, the diagnosis of BD-IPMN should be highly accurate to ensure that a pancreatic cyst chosen for surveillance is truly a BD-IPMN. Current diagnostic tools use imaging, clinical history, and cyst fluid analysis. While these can differentiate cyst types, there is enough overlap to raise diagnostic uncertainty. For example, a patient with a pancreatic cyst in the setting of pancreatitis is likely to have a pseudocyst (PC), a consequence of pancreatitis. In some cases, however, a pancreatic cyst, like a BD-IPMN, may be the cause of pancreatitis (Jang et al. 2013). Another example involves a mucinous cystic neoplasm (MCN). This typically presents as a solitary cyst in the pancreas body/tail of a middle-aged female. While this clinical profile suggests that the cyst is likely to be an MCN, the differential diagnosis includes a BD-IPMN. A final example involves serous cystadenomas (SCA). SCA lesions are benign non-mucinous cysts with characteristic imaging features that include a microcystic honeycomb appearance on imaging. Some SCAs, however, have an oligocystic appearance that can be difficult to discern from a BD-IPMN (Goh et al. 2006).

Thus, the ability to diagnose the histological subtype of pancreatic cyst based on clinical presentation, imaging, and clinical history is limited. With endoscopic ultrasound (EUS), cyst fluid aspiration for cytology and tumor marker analysis is relatively easy to perform; but this too has significant limitations. The lack of interpretable cells in the cyst fluid limits cytological analysis, providing a diagnostic sensitivity of 22 % for cancer and 35 % for premalignant mucinous cysts (Brugge et al. 2004). The tumor marker carcinoembryonic antigen (CEA) in cyst fluid can differentiate premalignant mucinous cysts with an area under the receiver operator curve (AUROC) of 0.79 (Brugge et al. 2004). Therefore, current diagnostic tools have less than ideal diagnostic accuracy leaving open the possibility that surveillance guidelines may be applied to some pancreatic cysts that are truly not BD-IPMN lesions.

The second ideal feature of a surveillance strategy would include having accurate biomarkers that diagnose the dysplasia status of a premalignant BD-IPMN. Knowing when high-grade dysplasia or noninvasive cancer evolves is the ultimate goal of current surveillance strategies. This “window of opportunity” is situated between missing invasive cancers when surgery is less effective as a treatment and removing a BD-IPMN prematurely when the risks of pancreatic surgery likely outweigh the benefit of cancer protection.

Current surveillance strategies have been developed without these ideal diagnostic tools using available clinical evidence and expert opinion. Should such tools be discovered, it has the potential to significantly change clinical practice and current surveillance methods. The following sections will describe the evolution and rationale of current surveillance methods.

11.3 Sendai Criteria 2006

In 2004, as part of a working group of the International Association of Pancreatology, a panel of physicians met to develop management guidelines for IPMNs and MCNs. They systematically reviewed the available evidence of pancreatic cystic neoplasms and proposed consensus-based criteria that were published in 2006 and are commonly referred to as the “Sendai criteria” (based on the meeting location in Japan) (Tanaka et al. 2006). They comprehensively addressed several clinical questions including (1) definitions and classification, (2) preoperative evaluation, (3) indication for resection, (4) methods of resection, (5) histological questions, and (6) methods of follow-up.

For the focus of this chapter, these criteria distinguished BD-IPMN from main duct IPMN (MD-IPMN) by imaging, histology, and clinical significance based on a synthesis of retrospective surgical series data demonstrating a difference in the prevalence of cancer. They reported a prevalence of cancer in MD-IPMN ranged from 57 % to 92 % and for BD-IPMN 6–46 % (Tanaka et al. 2006). This observation led the group to conclude that suspected MD-IPMN should be offered resection for surgically fit patients while suspected BD-IPMN could be monitored.

A distinction between MCN and IPMN was also made with clinical ramifications. It is postulated that MCN lesions arise from ovarian rests in the pancreas based on the presence of ovarian stroma in MCNs and the close histological and immunohistochemical resemblance to ovarian mucinous cystadenomas. This is in contrast to IPMNs, which arise from the pancreatic duct. MCNs are solitary lesions found in younger patients in the tail/body of the pancreas. In contrast BD-IPMNs are multifocal in up to 30 % of cases and occur more commonly in the head of the pancreas. The removal of MCNs requires the less morbid distal pancreatectomy, whereas a BD-IPMN in the head would require the more morbid pancreaticoduodenectomy. MCNs do not recur after surgical resection and patients therefore do not require post surgical surveillance. In contrast, additional BD-IPMNs may develop in the remnant pancreas after surgery thus requiring continued surveillance after surgical resection (Table 11.1).

While the risk of cancer in MCNs <4 cm is extremely low, for reasons noted above, it has been recommended that they be resected rather than be followed, potentially for decades. However, similar arguments could be made for an IPMN in a similar location in a young patient. Also, removal of an MCN in the neck of the pancreas could require removal of a significant portion of pancreas which could result in diabetes. Therefore, the decision to resect should weigh the risk and benefits of surgery, regardless of the predicted histological nature of cyst.

In contrast to recommending immediate resection for MD-IPMN, the rationale for observation of BD-IPMNs primarily stems from the low prevalence of cancer described above. Further review of these case series identified factors that predicted the absence of malignancy. Patients who had no correlating symptoms, a cyst size less than 3 cm, and no mural nodules had a very low probability of malignancy upon resection (Terris et al. 2000; Sugiyama et al. 2003; Matsumoto et al. 2003). Based on these limited studies, the working group concluded that while the decision to follow rather than resect a BD-IPMN is ultimately "a matter of clinical judgment," asymptomatic patients without main duct dilation (>6 mm), mural nodules, and cyst size less than 3 cm could be followed based on a low prevalence of cancer (0–5 %) and low risk of progression to invasive cancer over 12–36 months of follow-up.

Consequently, a surveillance algorithm for presumed BD-IPMNs was proposed and is reproduced in Fig. 11.1. Noninvasive imaging modalities including multidetector high-resolution computed tomography (CT) or magnetic resonance cholangiopancreatography (MRCP) were suggested as the primary means for surveillance, specifically looking for change in cyst size, change in main duct diameter, and development of intramural nodules. As a more invasive alternative, EUS can be used with a particular advantage in the assessment for intramural nodules. Based on opinion, the working group recommended annual follow-up for cysts less than 1 cm, 6–12 month follow-up for cysts between 1 and 2 cm, and 3–6 month follow-up for cysts greater than 2 cm. Cysts greater than 1 cm should consider obtaining an

Table 11.1 Key clinical and imaging differences between mucinous cystic neoplasms and branch-duct IPMNs

Cyst type	Age	Gender	Location	Cellular origin	Imaging appearance	Surgical resection	Postsurgical surveillance
Mucinous cystic neoplasm	50s	F>>M (95 % F)	Body/tail >> head	Unknown; suspect ovarian rest	Solitary cyst with occasional septations	Distal pancreatectomy	No
Branch-duct IPMN	70s	F=M	Head> body/tail	Pancreatic duct	Solitary or multifocal (~30 %), unilocular or multilocular	Often pancreaticoduodenectomy	Yes

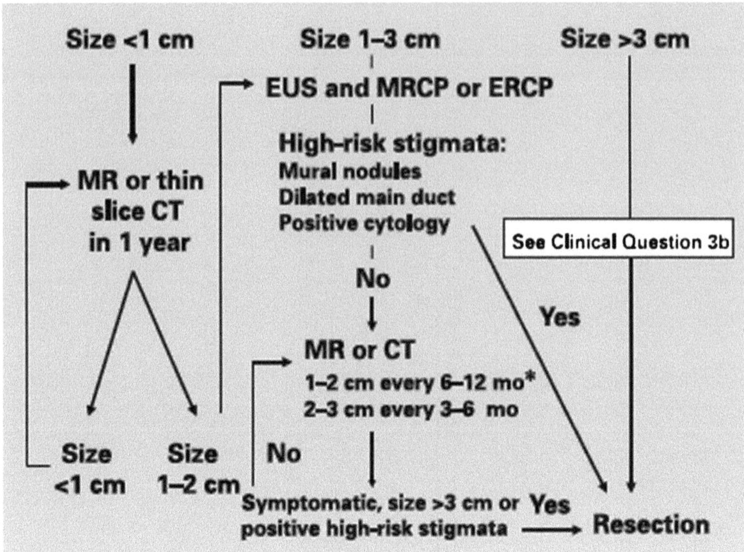

Fig. 11.1 First consensus algorithm for surveillance of branch-duct intraductal papillary mucinous neoplasms (a.k.a. Sendai criteria 2006). With permission from M. Tanaka

EUS to evaluate for intramural nodules and obtain cytology. The development of symptoms that correlate with the cyst (i.e., pancreatitis, jaundice, steatorrhea, unintentional weight loss), mural nodules, cyst greater than 3 cm, or dilation of the main duct beyond 6 mm during surveillance evaluation should warrant consideration for surgery.

For those BD-IPMNs that undergo resection, surveillance is still required. Invasive BD-IPMNs recur frequently (91 % in 3 years). Even in noninvasive BD-IPMNs, there is an estimated 8 % recurrence rate over 3 years of follow-up (Chari et al. 2002). Surveillance frequency with CT or MRI is recommended every 6 months for invasive BD-IPMNs and annually for noninvasive BD-IPMNs. The interval can be spaced out if there is no change over several years.

Several studies have evaluated the performance of these recommendations retrospectively. Paleaz-Luna and colleagues evaluated 77 BD-IPMNs with nine cancers and reported a sensitivity of 100 % and specificity of 23 % for diagnosing cancer using the Sendai criteria (Pelaez-Luna et al. 2007). Several other studies, some that specifically use the criteria and others that identified similar criteria to guide a selective approach, report similar results (Tang et al. 2008; Rodriguez et al. 2007; Salvia et al. 2007; Allen et al. 2006). The low specificity suggests that further refinement of the criteria may help minimize unnecessary surgical resections. In particular, the use of size as a criterion for surgical resection has been questioned. In a large single-center outcomes study by Walsh and colleagues, they reported that using size in asymptomatic patients subjected 28 % of asymptomatic patients with cysts greater than 3 cm to unnecessary surgery (Walsh et al. 2008).

Correa-Gallego and colleagues performed a single-center study that correlated pre- and postoperative diagnosis of incidentally discovered cysts that were operated on immediately ($n=136$) or after an initial period of observation ($n=23$) based on Sendai criteria (Correa-Gallego et al. 2010). The preoperative diagnosis was incorrect in 32 % of the cases in the immediate surgery group and 48 % of the cases in the observation group. Approximately 5 % of patients who had a benign nonneoplastic cyst underwent surgery. Another source of preoperative misdiagnosis involved distinguishing MCN from BD-IPMN. This study highlights the limitations of current imaging and surveillance methods and the need to develop better tests to detect high-risk premalignant BD-IPMNs. While there were substantial discrepancies between radiographic and histological diagnosis, the Sendai criteria of 2006 performed reasonably well but clearly needed refinement.

11.4 Fukuoka Criteria 2012

With increasing recognition of BD-IPMNs and MCNs, another symposium under the auspices of the International Association of Pancreatology was held in Fukuoka, Japan in 2010 (Tanaka et al. 2012). This brought together a larger panel of physicians to consider new data since 2004 with the intent to revise the Sendai criteria. Despite more data, the panel maintained the guidelines as "consensus based" (in contrast to evidence based) given the overall low quality of evidence. Regarding changes related to BD-IPMN, the accumulation of data since the Sendai criteria supports a strategy of "deliberate observation" over "early resection."

Since the frequency of malignancy in BD-IPMN was first summarized in the Sendai criteria report (6–46 %), there have been several subsequent studies included for consideration in the Fukuoka meeting. In a pooled analysis, of these studies, a total of 2027 BD-IPMNs were described with malignancy reported in 6–51 % of cases and invasive cancers reported in 1–37 % of cases (Tanaka et al. 2012). Among these studies, the largest contribution of BD-IPMNs came from multicenter retrospective study in Japan by Suzuki and colleagues (Suzuki et al. 2004). This study reported on 509 surgically verified BD-IPMNs with a mean diameter of 27.3 ± 15.9 mm and reported a prevalence of invasive cancer of 29.5 %. Four studies from the United States, Italy, Japan, and South Korea focused only on BD-IPMNs with the frequency of malignancy ranging between 8 % and 25 % and invasive cancer between 1.4 % and 12 % (Rodriguez et al. 2007; Jang et al. 2008; Sadakari et al. 2010; Kanno et al. 2010). While the study by Rodriguez and colleagues (Rodriguez et al. 2007) and Sadakari and colleagues (Sadakari et al. 2010) found no malignancies less than 3 cm, Jang and colleagues (Jang et al. 2008) observed a tumor size of >2 cm to be the most valuable predictor of malignancy.

The frequency estimate of malignancy in BD-IPMN has changed little since the Sendai criteria and remains significant enough to consider surgical resection. There are reasons, again, to prompt caution for immediate surgery. First, it is important to remember that the vast majority of these studies came from retrospective surgical series, which likely overestimate the frequency of malignancy. Second, BD-IPMNs are more frequently observed in the elderly (~9 %), who have competing risks of mortality including increased complications from surgical resection. Third, the low estimated annual malignancy conversion rate of approximately 1 % still makes an observation strategy more favorable for many patients (Al-Haddad et al. 2011; Khannoussi et al. 2012). And fourth, the current monitoring approach by the Sendai criteria has been validated by several studies (Pelaez-Luna et al. 2007; Tang et al. 2008; Rodriguez et al. 2007; Salvia et al. 2007; Allen et al. 2006).

Expanding upon the Sendai criteria, the Fukuoka criteria attempts to risk-stratify clinical and imaging variables to be more selective of patients who would benefit from immediate resection. Patients with (1) obstructive jaundice, (2) an enhanced solid component, or (3) a main pancreatic diameter size of greater than 10 mm have "high-risk stigmata" and should undergo immediate resection without further testing. Another group of variables includes a BD-IPMN that (1) is greater than 3 cm, (2) has thickened enhanced cyst walls, (3) has a main pancreatic duct dilation of 5–9 mm, (4) has a non-enhanced mural nodule, (5) has an abrupt change in main pancreatic duct caliber with distal pancreatic atrophy, (6) has lymphadenopathy, and (7) is associated with pancreatitis, which are labeled "worrisome features." These findings, when present, warrant further investigation with EUS. The recommendation to not proceed to surgery for BD-IPMNs greater than 3 cm, the presence of any mural nodule, or a dilated main duct greater than 6 mm represents a clear change from the Sendai criteria.

In the Fukuoka criteria, the primary role of EUS is to further evaluate pancreatic cysts with worrisome features and for cysts greater than 2 cm under surveillance. Specifically, EUS can better define a mural nodule seen on CT or MRI/MRCP. The presence of Doppler flow and lack of mobility suggest a true neoplastic nodule that should be confirmed by fine needle aspiration (FNA). Mobile non-enhancing "mural nodules" are likely conglomerates of mucin that EUS should be able to discriminate. EUS can also be used to further evaluate the main duct involvement that is suggested by the presence of thickened ductal walls, intraductal mucin, or mural nodules within the main pancreatic duct. EUS can be used to aspirate cyst fluid as well as mural nodules for cytology and, if suspicious or positive for malignancy, facilitate the decision to offer surgery.

Although the role of EUS is limited, it has the most potential to transform current clinical practice of BD-IPMNs. The pancreatic cyst is a relatively protected space comprised of secreted biological material from the epithelial cyst lining that is easily obtainable by FNA. Current cyst fluid biomarkers like CEA, however, have little impact on surgical decision-making, except when differentiating an oligocystic SCA from a BD-IPMN or MCN (Goh et al. 2006; Brugge et al. 2004; Cohen-Scali et al. 2003; Kim et al. 2006). Novel cyst fluid biomarkers have garnered significant interest in the past 5 years that include studying differences in detectable DNA, proteins, inflammatory cytokines, and micro RNA in the cyst fluid (Allen et al. 2009; Haab et al. 2010; Maker et al. 2011; Ryu et al. 2011; Wu et al. 2011; Khalid et al. 2009; Shen et al. 2009).

Furthermore, refinements in cytological interpretation may also increase the utility of EUS. Previous reports on the diagnostic utility of cytology for BD-IPMNs were poor because the amount of obtained cellular material was qualitatively and quantitatively insufficient for malignant interpretation. The use of "high-grade epithelial atypia" which identifies cellular atypia without meeting the requirements for a malignancy diagnosis has demonstrated clinical value. In one study, the use of this classification had 72 % sensitivity for diagnosing malignancy within a mucinous cyst (Pitman et al. 2010). In another study, the use of "high-grade epithelial atypia" detected 30 % more cancers in small BD-IPMNs (Genevay et al. 2011).

One aspect of EUS with FNA that has limited its enthusiasm and potential is the concern that FNA-related leakage of cyst fluid contents can lead to peritoneal dissemination (Hirooka et al. 2003). Further evidence to support this concern is needed. Although the promises of EUS are acknowledged in the Fukuoka criteria, the working group concluded that EUS-FNA for cytological and molecular analysis remains investigational and should be limited to centers with expertise pending further data.

Like the Sendai criteria, the Fukuoka criteria conclude that there is "little evidence in the literature to guide the frequency and type of surveillance for IPMNs" and that the decision is ultimately a matter of clinical judgment. Prior to considering surveillance, a baseline history, physical examination, and MRI/MRCP (or CT) should be performed. Consistent with a recent consensus of radiologists, the working group recommended gadolinium-enhanced MRI with MRCP as a preferred imaging modality for investigating and monitoring BD-IPMN lesions (Berland et al. 2010). Gadolinium-enhanced MRI with MRCP offers superior contrast resolution to facilitate recognition of cyst septae, nodules, and duct communication and avoid radiation exposure.

Once the initial investigation is complete, patients with high-risk stigmata who are surgically fit should be offered surgery. Patients with worrisome features should be offered EUS for further risk stratification. Should no evidence of a definite mural nodule, main duct involvement, or cytology suspicious for malignancy be present on EUS, a recommendation for surveillance can be made. When there is no prior imaging, a short interval follow-up at 3–6 months with MRI/MRCP or CT is recommended to establish cyst stability. Subsequent surveillance is based on cyst size as summarized in Fig. 11.2.

For BD-IPMNs less than 1 cm, an MRI/MRCP or CT is recommended every 2–3 years, which represents a lengthening of the frequency interval from the Sendai criteria. For BD-IPMNs between 1 and 2 cm, yearly MRI/MRCP or CT is recommended for 2 years. If there is no change observed, then extending the interval is recommended but no clear guidance from the working group is explicitly provided. For BD-IPMNs between 2 and 3 cm, EUS is recommended in 3–6 months, and then lengthening the interval is appropriate alternating between MRI/MRCP and EUS. Again, the working group provides no clear guidance as to the lengthening of the interval. For those cysts greater than 3 cm, alternating between MRI/MRCP and EUS is recommended every 3–6 months. For cysts greater than 2 cm in young (less than 65) surgically fit patients, it may be more beneficial to consider surgery instead of a prolonged surveillance strategy.

These imprecise recommendations for surveillance frequency are based on several considerations. First, there is a lack of data that supports the safety of lengthening out the monitoring interval to 2 years. Several reports of pancreatic

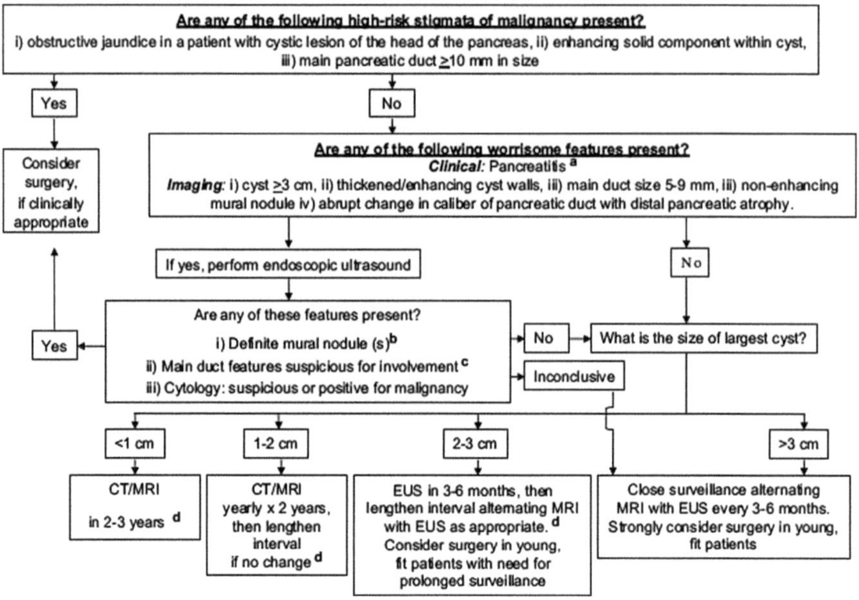

Fig. 11.2 Second consensus algorithm for surveillance of branch-duct intraductal papillary mucinous neoplasms (a.k.a. Fukuoka criteria 2012). With permission from M. Tanaka

cancer development in patients with BD-IPMN have prompted some investigators to advocate for 6-month interval surveillance regardless of cyst size (Tada et al. 2006; Tanno et al. 2010a; Tanno et al. 2010b). Second, there is a lack of data to support discontinuation of surveillance after a period of undefined long-term stability. Third, one small study suggests that a rapid growth rate (greater than 2 mm per year) correlates with increasing risk of malignancy, which would require the flexibility to shorten the interval of surveillance (Kang et al. 2011). Finally, BD-IPMNs manifest a field defect leading to a higher risk of developing pancreatic cancer anywhere in the pancreas. This makes shorter intervals more appealing and lengthening or discontinuing surveillance less so. More natural history data is sorely needed.

For those BD-IPMNs that undergo surgical resection, the follow-up strategy depends on certain circumstances. In the case of multifocal IPMN where known BD-IPMNs remain in the remnant pancreas, the method of surveillance and frequency should follow the algorithm of non-resected BD-IPMNs. For those without remnant BD-IPMNs, follow-up includes repeat imaging with MRI/MRCP or CT in 2 and 5 years based on available evidence that suggests a recurrence rate between 0 % and 20 % at 5 years (Chari et al. 2002; White et al. 2007). As noted above, a more conservative surveillance strategy may involve repeated imaging every 6 months in light of an estimated 0.9 % annual risk of distinct pancreatic adenocarcinoma development (Tada et al. 2006; Tanno et al. 2010a; Tanno et al. 2010b).

Extrapolating from the relationship of family history and established genetic defects and pancreatic adenocarcinoma, the risk of a BD-IPMN in the context of a strong family history (two or more first degree relatives with pancreatic cancer) may entail a stronger risk of cancer development prompting a more aggressive surveillance strategy. The working group recommends an MRI/MRCP or CT and EUS for initial assessment of high-risk stigmata and worrisome features. Presence of any of these features warrants resection for those surgically fit. If these features are absent, surveillance with MRI/MRCP or CT every 3 months with annual EUS for 2 years is recommended. Development of worrisome features should prompt immediate surgical resection. It is important to highlight that these recommendations are based on consensus among the working group panel with little to no supporting direct evidence.

Beyond surveillance of the development of pancreatic cancer among non-resected BD-IPMN and the remnant pancreas from resected BD-IPMN, there is also an association between BD-IPMN and synchronous and metachronous extrapancreatic benign neoplasms and cancers with an estimated incidence of 10–50 % (Sugiyama and Atomi 1999; Benarroch-Gampel and Riall 2010). In one large case–control study by Reid-Lombardo and colleagues, 471 cases of IPMN were compared to 471 patients with pancreatic adenocarcinoma and 1,413 patients in the general population. The proportion of extrapancreatic neoplasms diagnosed before or at the time of IPMN diagnosis was 52 % (95 % CI, 47–56 %), compared with 36 % (95 % CI, 32–41 %) in patients with pancreatic adenocarcinoma ($P<0.001$), and 43 % (95 % CI, 41–46 %) in the general population ($P=0.002$). The most frequent benign neoplasms included colon polyps and Barrett's esophagus, and the most frequent cancers included nonmelanoma skin, breast, prostate, and carcinoid cancers (Reid-Lombardo et al. 2010). In Asian populations, colon polyps and cancers were also observed in addition to gastric cancer (Sugiyama and Atomi 1999). At this time, no established screening or surveillance guidelines exist.

11.5 Conclusion

Frequent use of high-resolution CT and MRI imaging has given emergence to asymptomatic (and symptomatic) pancreatic cysts of which BD-IPMNs represent one of the most common premalignant neoplastic conditions. From routine surgical resection that characterized clinical practice in the 1990s, a surveillance approach has evolved that attempts to balance the risks and benefits between pancreatic cancer progression and surgical resection. The lack of a minimally invasive and safe technique to acquire cyst wall tissue for diagnosis has given rise to a preoperative consensus-based surveillance approach using clinical and imaging characteristics. The first algorithm (a.k.a. Sendai criteria) was published in 2006 and demonstrated great sensitivity but poor specificity for guiding surgical treatment for malignancy.

A recent revision to this algorithm, the Fukuoka criteria, published in 2012, expands upon the first algorithm to attempt to raise the specificity. In these criteria, patients with high-risk stigmata associated with BD-IPMN should undergo immediate resection for those surgically fit. High-risk stigmata include obstructive jaundice, an enhancing mural nodule, or main duct involvement greater than 10 mm. Patients with worrisome features should undergo an EUS. Worrisome features include a cyst size greater than 3 cm, main duct dilation between 5 and 9 mm, thickened cyst wall, non-enhancing mural nodule, associated pancreatitis, abrupt change in main duct caliber with pancreatic atrophy, and lymphadenopathy. If EUS confirms a mural nodule, main duct involvement, or suspicious cytology, then surgery is indicated. If not, surveillance is recommended stratified by cyst size with consideration for proceeding to surgery for those younger patients whom prolonged surveillance is less attractive.

While bringing together international consensus is important to standardize and disseminate clinical practice for surveillance of BD-IPMNs, many of these recommendations lack direct evidence. Improvements in surveillance will hinge on continued, concentrated research into the natural history of BD-IPMNs as well as into its biology to develop appropriate serum or cyst fluid-based biomarkers for accurate diagnosis and prognosis.

References

Adsay NV. Cystic lesions of the pancreas. Mod Pathol. 2007;20 Suppl 1:S71–93.

Al-Haddad M, Schmidt MC, Sandrasegaran K, et al. Diagnosis and treatment of cystic pancreatic tumors. Clin Gastroenterol Hepatol. 2011;9:635–48.

Allen PJ, D'Angelica M, Gonen M, et al. A selective approach to the resection of cystic lesions of the pancreas: results from 539 consecutive patients. Ann Surg. 2006;244:572–82.

Allen PJ, Qin LX, Tang L, et al. Pancreatic cyst fluid protein expression profiling for discriminating between serous cystadenoma and intraductal papillary mucinous neoplasm. Ann Surg. 2009; 250:754–60.

Benarroch-Gampel J, Riall TS. Extrapancreatic malignancies and intraductal papillary mucinous neoplasms of the pancreas. World J Gastrointest Surg. 2010;2:363–7.

Berland LL, Silverman SG, Gore RM, et al. Managing incidental findings on abdominal CT: white paper of the ACR incidental findings committee. J Am Coll Radiol. 2010;7:754–73.

Brugge WR, Lewandrowski K, Lee-Lewandrowski E, et al. Diagnosis of pancreatic cystic neoplasms: a report of the cooperative pancreatic cyst study. Gastroenterology. 2004;126:1330–6.

Chari ST, Yadav D, Smyrk TC, et al. Study of recurrence after surgical resection of intraductal papillary mucinous neoplasm of the pancreas. Gastroenterology. 2002;123:1500–7.

Cohen-Scali F, Vilgrain V, Brancatelli G, et al. Discrimination of unilocular macrocystic serous cystadenoma from pancreatic pseudocyst and mucinous cystadenoma with CT: initial observations. Radiology. 2003;228:727–33.

Correa-Gallego C, Ferrone CR, Thayer SP, et al. Incidental pancreatic cysts: do we really know what we are watching? Pancreatology. 2010;10:144–50.

de Jong K, Nio CY, Hermans JJ, Dijkgraaf MG, Gouma DJ, van Eijck CHJ, et al. Prevalence of pancreatic cysts in individuals undergoing preventive medical examination by magnetic resonance imaging (MRI). Clin Gastroenterol Hepatol. 2010;8.

Genevay M, Mino-Kenudson M, Yaeger K, et al. Cytology adds value to imaging studies for risk assessment of malignancy in pancreatic mucinous cysts. Ann Surg. 2011;254:977–83.

Goh BK, Tan YM, Yap WM, et al. Pancreatic serous oligocystic adenomas: clinicopathologic features and a comparison with serous microcystic adenomas and mucinous cystic neoplasms. World J Surg. 2006;30:1553–9.

Haab BB, Porter A, Yue T, et al. Glycosylation variants of mucins and CEACAMs as candidate biomarkers for the diagnosis of pancreatic cystic neoplasms. Ann Surg. 2010;251:937–45.

Hirooka Y, Goto H, Itoh A, et al. Case of intraductal papillary mucinous tumor in which endosonography-guided fine-needle aspiration biopsy caused dissemination. J Gastroenterol Hepatol. 2003;18:1323–4.

Howlader NNA, Krapcho M, Neyman N, et al., editors. SEER cancer statistics review, 1975–2009 (Vintage 2009 populations). Bethesda: National Cancer Institute; 2012.

Jang JY, Kim SW, Lee SE, et al. Treatment guidelines for branch duct type intraductal papillary mucinous neoplasms of the pancreas: when can we operate or observe? Ann Surg Oncol. 2008;15:199–205.

Jang JW, Kim MH, Jeong SU, et al. Clinical characteristics of IPMN manifesting as acute pancreatitis or acute recurrent pancreatitis. J Gastroenterol Hepatol. 2013;28(4):731–8.

Kang MJ, Jang JY, Kim SJ, et al. Cyst growth rate predicts malignancy in patients with branch duct intraductal papillary mucinous neoplasms. Clin Gastroenterol Hepatol. 2011;9:87–93.

Kanno A, Satoh K, Hirota M, et al. Prediction of invasive carcinoma in branch type intraductal papillary mucinous neoplasms of the pancreas. J Gastroenterol. 2010;45:952–9.

Khalid A, Zahid M, Finkelstein SD, et al. Pancreatic cyst fluid DNA analysis in evaluating pancreatic cysts: a report of the PANDA study. Gastrointest Endosc. 2009;69:1095–102.

Khannoussi W, Vullierme MP, Rebours V, et al. The long term risk of malignancy in patients with branch duct intraductal papillary mucinous neoplasms of the pancreas. Pancreatology. 2012;12:198–202.

Kim SY, Lee JM, Kim SH, et al. Macrocystic neoplasms of the pancreas: CT differentiation of serous oligocystic adenoma from mucinous cystadenoma and intraductal papillary mucinous tumor. AJR Am J Roentgenol. 2006;187:1192–8.

Laffan TA, Horton KM, Klein AP, et al. Prevalence of unsuspected pancreatic cysts on MDCT. AJR Am J Roentgenol. 2008;191:802–7.

Maker AV, Katabi N, Qin LX, et al. Cyst fluid interleukin-1β (IL1β) levels predict the risk of carcinoma in intraductal papillary mucinous neoplasms of the pancreas. Clin Cancer Res. 2011;17:1502–8.

Matsumoto T, Aramaki M, Yada K, et al. Optimal management of the branch duct type intraductal papillary mucinous neoplasms of the pancreas. J Clin Gastroenterol. 2003;36:261–5.

McPhee JT, Hill JS, Whalen GF, et al. Perioperative mortality for pancreatectomy: a national perspective. Ann Surg. 2007;246:246–53.

Pelaez-Luna M, Chari ST, Smyrk TC, et al. Do consensus indications for resection in branch duct intraductal papillary mucinous neoplasm predict malignancy? A study of 147 patients. Am J Gastroenterol. 2007;102:1759–64.

Pitman MB, Genevay M, Yaeger K, et al. High-grade atypical epithelial cells in pancreatic mucinous cysts are a more accurate predictor of malignancy than "positive" cytology. Cancer Cytopathol. 2010;118:434–40.

Reid-Lombardo KM, Mathis KL, Wood CM, et al. Frequency of extrapancreatic neoplasms in intraductal papillary mucinous neoplasm of the pancreas: implications for management. Ann Surg. 2010;251:64–9.

Rodriguez JR, Salvia R, Crippa S, et al. Branch-duct intraductal papillary mucinous neoplasms: observations in 145 patients who underwent resection. Gastroenterology. 2007;133:72–9. quiz 309–10.

Ryu JK, Matthaei H, Dal Molin M, et al. Elevated microRNA miR-21 levels in pancreatic cyst fluid are predictive of mucinous precursor lesions of ductal adenocarcinoma. Pancreatology. 2011;11:343–50.

Sadakari Y, Ienaga J, Kobayashi K, et al. Cyst size indicates malignant transformation in branch duct intraductal papillary mucinous neoplasm of the pancreas without mural nodules. Pancreas. 2010;39:232–6.

Salvia R, Crippa S, Falconi M, et al. Branch-duct intraductal papillary mucinous neoplasms of the pancreas: to operate or not to operate? Gut. 2007;56:1086–90.

Shen J, Brugge WR, Dimaio CJ, et al. Molecular analysis of pancreatic cyst fluid: a comparative analysis with current practice of diagnosis. Cancer. 2009;117:217–27.

Sugiyama M, Atomi Y. Extrapancreatic neoplasms occur with unusual frequency in patients with intraductal papillary mucinous tumors of the pancreas. Am J Gastroenterol. 1999;94:470–3.

Sugiyama M, Izumisato Y, Abe N, et al. Predictive factors for malignancy in intraductal papillary-mucinous tumours of the pancreas. Br J Surg. 2003;90:1244–9.
Suzuki Y, Atomi Y, Sugiyama M, et al. Cystic neoplasm of the pancreas: a Japanese multiinstitutional study of intraductal papillary mucinous tumor and mucinous cystic tumor. Pancreas. 2004;28:241–6.
Tada M, Kawabe T, Arizumi M, et al. Pancreatic cancer in patients with pancreatic cystic lesions: a prospective study in 197 patients. Clin Gastroenterol Hepatol. 2006;4:1265–70.
Tanaka M, Chari S, Adsay V, et al. International consensus guidelines for management of intraductal papillary mucinous neoplasms and mucinous cystic neoplasms of the pancreas. Pancreatology. 2006;6:17–32.
Tanaka M, Fernandez-Del Castillo C, Adsay V, et al. International consensus guidelines 2012 for the management of IPMN and MCN of the pancreas. Pancreatology. 2012;12:183–97.
Tang RS, Weinberg B, Dawson DW, et al. Evaluation of the guidelines for management of pancreatic branch-duct intraductal papillary mucinous neoplasm. Clin Gastroenterol Hepatol. 2008;6:815–9. quiz 719.
Tanno S, Nakano Y, Koizumi K, et al. Pancreatic ductal adenocarcinomas in long-term follow-up patients with branch duct intraductal papillary mucinous neoplasms. Pancreas. 2010a;39:36–40.
Tanno S, Nakano Y, Sugiyama Y, et al. Incidence of synchronous and metachronous pancreatic carcinoma in 168 patients with branch duct intraductal papillary mucinous neoplasm. Pancreatology. 2010b;10:173–8.
Terris B, Ponsot P, Paye F, et al. Intraductal papillary mucinous tumors of the pancreas confined to secondary ducts show less aggressive pathologic features as compared with those involving the main pancreatic duct. Am J Surg Pathol. 2000;24:1372–7.
Venkat R, Edil BH, Schulick RD, et al. Laparoscopic distal pancreatectomy is associated with significantly less overall morbidity compared to the open technique: a systematic review and meta-analysis. Ann Surg. 2012;255:1048–59.
Walsh RM, Vogt DP, Henderson JM, et al. Management of suspected pancreatic cystic neoplasms based on cyst size. Surgery. 2008;144:677–84. discussion 684–5.
White R, D'Angelica M, Katabi N, et al. Fate of the remnant pancreas after resection of noninvasive intraductal papillary mucinous neoplasm. J Am Coll Surg. 2007;204:987–93. discussion 993–5.
Wu J, Matthaei H, Maitra A, et al. Recurrent GNAS mutations define an unexpected pathway for pancreatic cyst development. Sci Transl Med. 2011;3:92ra66.

Part IV
Management

Chapter 12
Timing of Resection of Main-Duct IPMN

Klaus Sahora and Carlos Fernández-del Castillo

Abstract Considering the high prevalence of malignancy in MD-IPMN, the international consensus guidelines for the management of IPMN and MCN of the pancreas recommend surgical resection of MD-IPMN for all surgically fit patients. The extent and type of preoperative work-up in patients with MD-IPMN should be orientated on the nature of the presenting symptoms, the certainty of the diagnosis, the likelihood that malignancy is present, and the age and surgical risk of the patient. In frail patients a primary observational approach, until the onset of symptoms or the appearance of findings suspicious for malignancy, may be a compromise strategy. A standard pancreaticoduodenectomy or distal pancreatectomy is the procedure of choice. However, it is important that patients have been preoperatively informed, not only about the extent of the planned procedure but also about the probability of an extended resection going as far as a total pancreatectomy.

Keywords Cystic neoplasm • Intraductal papillary mucinous neoplasm • Pancreas • Surgery

12.1 Introduction

The natural history of intraductal papillary mucinous neoplasms (IPMN) has been intensively studied within the last 20 years, and many new insights have been gained since then. Based on the involvement of the main pancreatic duct and its tributaries,

K. Sahora
Department of Surgery, Medical University of Vienna,
Waehringer Gvertel 18–20, Vienna 1010, Austria

C. Fernández-del Castillo (✉)
Wang Ambulatory Care Center, Massachusetts General Hospital,
15 Parkman Street, Boston, MA 02114, USA
e-mail: CFERNANDEZ@partners.org

M. Tanaka (ed.), *Intraductal Papillary Mucinous Neoplasm of the Pancreas*,
DOI 10.1007/978-4-431-54472-2_12, © Springer Japan 2014

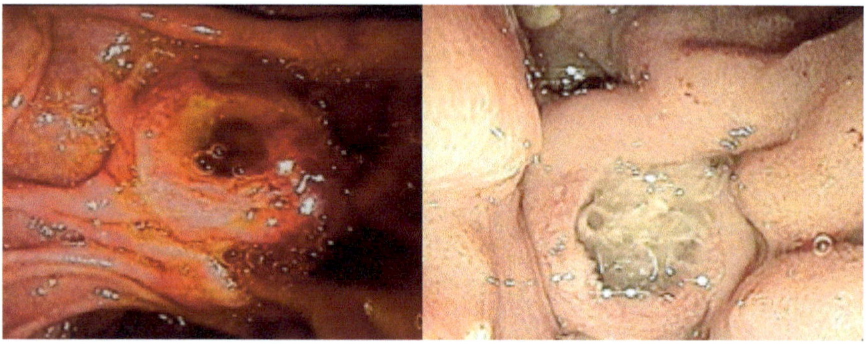

Fig. 12.1 Two typical endoscopic views of a bulging ampulla

IPMN are categorized as main-duct, branch-duct, and combined IPMN. According to the degree of epithelial dysplasia, they are moreover classified as adenoma (low-grade dysplasia), borderline (moderate dysplasia), carcinoma in situ (high-grade dysplasia), and invasive carcinoma. In its classic form, main-duct IPMN presents as a dilated main pancreatic duct (MD-IPMN), full of mucus that extrudes through a bulging ampulla (Fig. 12.1). Today it is without any controversy that over time MD-IPMN follow an adenoma-carcinoma sequence and transform into invasive adenocarcinoma. In large surgical series the rate of malignancy found in MD-IPMN is ~60 % (36–100 %) and the rate of invasive cancer is ~43 % (11–81 %) (Salvia et al. 2004; Suzuki et al. 2004; Crippa et al. 2010). MD-IPMN do present with a slight predominance in elderly male patients (~65 years), and patients with malignant MD-IPMN are commonly older (~6 years) than those with benign lesions (Salvia et al. 2010; Fernandez-Del Castillo and Adsay 2010). Based on the natural course of MD-IPMN, a surgical approach is recommended in most patients (Tanaka et al. 2006, 2012).

12.2 Indication for Resection of Main-Duct IPMN

Considering the high prevalence of malignancy in MD-IPMN, the international consensus guidelines for the management of IPMN and MCN of the pancreas recommend surgical resection of MD-IPMN for all surgically fit patients (Tanaka et al. 2006, 2012). The rationale for resection is: (1) to ameliorate symptoms, (2) to remove lesions at high risk for malignant transformation, and (3) to potentially cure invasive lesions. However, in a subset of patients with high surgical risk or with competing life-terminating conditions (i.e., other malignancies), it is reasonable to pursue an observational approach. Some authors furthermore described that there is a subset of MD-IPMN with a lower likelihood of progression into malignancy and in analogy to branch-duct IPMN, these could be treated by close observation (Takuma et al. 2011; Uehara et al. 2010). The 2012 revised international guidelines define these "low-risk" MD-IPMN as MPD dilation of 5–9 mm without any other worrisome feature (i.e., presence of symptoms or mural nodules/mass) and evaluation, but no immediate resection is recommended for selected patients. Data on such conservative approach is extremely limited and mainly includes patients with an obvious high risk of surgical morbidity and mortality. Uehara et al. defined MD-IPMN with lower likelihood of malignancy as follows: a main pancreatic duct diameter of less than 10 mm, no visualized mural nodule, and a negative result of the cytological examination of pancreatic juice (Uehara et al. 2010). In that series of 20 observed low-risk MD-IPMN, with a mean follow-up of 70 months, two patients progressed beyond low-risk criteria and underwent resection with the final diagnosis of invasive MD-IPMN carcinoma in one and carcinoma in situ in the second patient. The author concluded that selected MD-IPMN can be followed by close observation as long as low-risk criteria are fulfilled. Another small series published by Takuma et al. described the outcome of 20 patients with MD-IPMN, who have been conservatively followed because of a high surgical risk related to major comorbidities (Takuma et al. 2011). After a median follow-up of 48 months, nine patients (45 %) died from their comorbidities, 3 (15 %) died of pancreatic cancer, and one patient was alive with documented conversion into pancreatic cancer. Of note, all patients who progressed into cancer demonstrated an increment of main pancreatic duct diameter.

12.3 Preoperative Diagnosis and Work-up

The extent and type of preoperative work-up in patients with MD-IPMN should be orientated on the nature of the presenting symptoms, the certainty of the diagnosis, the likelihood that malignancy is present, and the age and surgical risk of the patient.

Pancreatic protocol CT or gadolinium-enhanced MRI gives very precise information on the type, location, and extent of the tumor. Both modalities are comparable in detecting associated masses, adjacent organ infiltration, and lymph node or organ metastases. MRI is the procedure of choice by many radiologists, being superior in the recognition of septae and nodules. In addition magnetic resonance cholangiopancreatography (MRCP) provides a noninvasive way to assess the biliary and pancreatic ducts (Fig. 12.2). Enhancing of the pancreatic duct wall, the degree of duct dilation, and the presence of a mural nodule or associated mass are commonly reported findings for malignant MD-IPMN (Manfredi et al. 2009; Sugiyama et al. 2003).

The use of endoscopic ultrasound (EUS) with fine-needle aspiration (FNA) in the diagnosis of MD-IPMN can help to assess the extent of involvement and in detecting small nodules or an associated mass (Ohno et al. 2011). In high-risk patients, preoperative tissue diagnosis by FNA and confirmation of malignancy may be helpful in making the decision for or against surgery.

Endoscopic retrograde cholangiopancreatography (ERCP) has widely been displaced by MRCP and is no longer routine for the evaluation of these patients. When done, ERCP may disclose a pathognomonic bulging papilla with a patulous

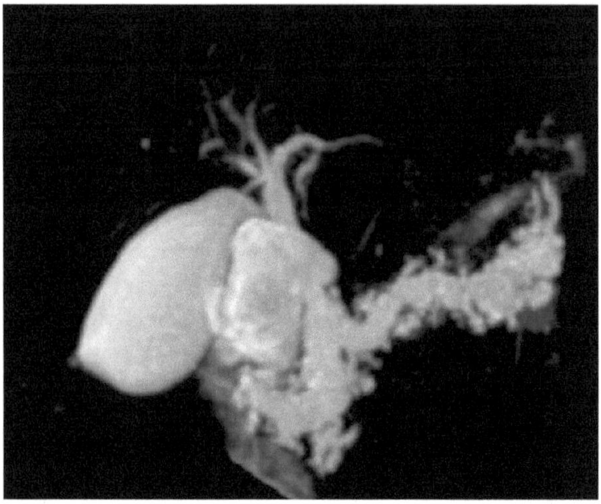

Fig. 12.2 MRCP of an IPMN, diffuse type, combined main and branch-duct type

orifice extruding mucus (Aso et al. 2012). According to the 2012 IAP guidelines, routine ERCP for sampling of fluid or brushings in IPMN is no longer recommended (Tanaka et al. 2006, 2012).

12.4 Timing of Resection of Main-Duct IPMN

All surgically fit patients diagnosed with MD-IPMN should undergo resection in the foreseeable future. In patients with MD-IPMN not showing worrisome morphological features or major symptoms, surgery might be scheduled more amply within several months, while patients with lesions harboring a high risk for malignancy should undergo immediate surgery. In frail patients a primary observational approach, until the onset of symptoms or the appearance of findings suspicious for malignancy, may be a compromise strategy.

12.5 Method of Resection of Main-Duct IPMN

Determination of the appropriate surgical strategy in MD-IPMN can be challenging. First, in contrast to other pancreatic neoplasms where a pancreatic mass is obvious, MD-IPMN commonly present as diffuse dilation of the main pancreatic duct (Fig. 12.3), often without an associated pancreatic mass. This dilation may be caused by MD-IPMN, which can spread along the entire duct, but it might also

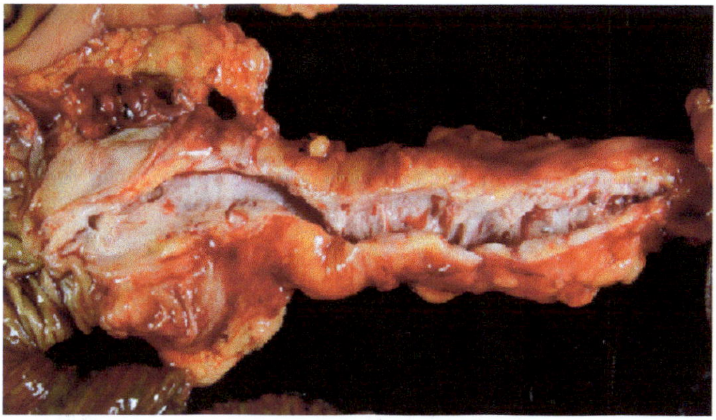

Fig. 12.3 Diffuse MD-IPMN involving the entire gland

occur because of overproduction of mucus and/or associated chronic pancreatitis, making location problematic. Second, involvement of the main pancreatic duct can range from focal to diffuse, including skip lesions of normal ductal epithelium. In this setting the surgeon has to determine the appropriate segment of resection and type of resection but has to be aware to change his strategy if needed. Therefore, it is important that patients have been preoperatively informed, not only about the extent of the planned procedure but also about the probability of an extended resection going as far as a total pancreatectomy.

This obviously needs to be individualized carefully. Whereas a total pancreatectomy may be appropriate in a young, fit patient who has an IPMN with carcinoma in the head of the pancreas that is extending into the body and tail, it may not be the right operation for an elderly or frail patient with an IPMN that is only an adenoma or borderline tumor, even if present at the transection margin.

In general, in the segmental ectatic-type MD-IPMN (Fig. 12.4) or diffuse type with focal lesions, a standard pancreaticoduodenectomy or distal pancreatectomy is the procedure of choice. In our experience with 229 patients with IPMN involving the main pancreatic duct (52 MD-IPMN, 172 combined IPMN), 65 % have required a Whipple resection, 10 % a total pancreatectomy, 23 % a distal pancreatectomy, and 2 % of patients resection of the middle segment of the pancreas. The overall mortality in our series was 1 %.

12.5.1 Lymphadenectomy

Pancreatectomy with lymph node dissection remains the standard treatment for invasive MD-IPMN carcinoma. Resections without lymphadenectomy should only be considered in patients where malignancy is very unlikely or has been ruled out.

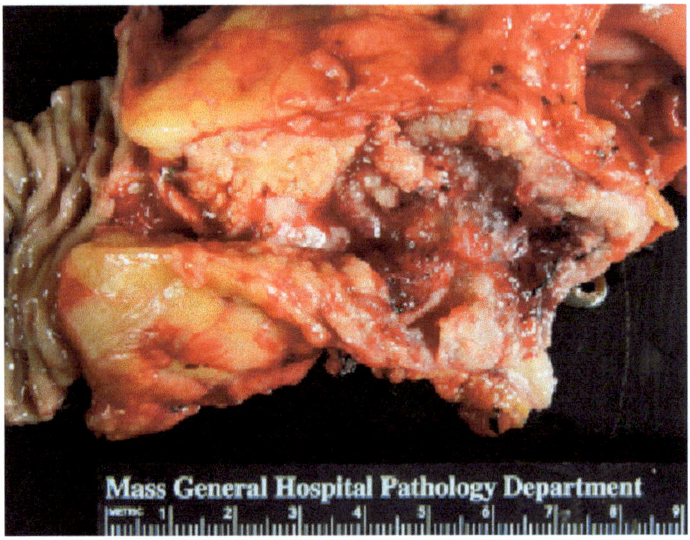

Fig. 12.4 Segmental ectatic-type MD-IPMN with typical intraductal papillary proliferations

12.5.2 Transection Margin and Frozen Section

Because MD-IPMN extends along the pancreatic duct and can do so without obvious macroscopic tumor, it is important to rule out presence of tumor in the margin so as not to leave tumor behind. A denuded epithelium within the duct is not uncommon in this pathology, and de-epithelialization should not erroneously be interpreted as a "negative" margin, because recurrence has occurred in this setting. Frozen sections during resection are useful for deciding the resection line (Couvelard et al. 2005).

According the international guidelines, if the resection margin is positive for IPMN with high-grade dysplasia, additional resection of the pancreas should be attempted to obtain a negative margin. In the case of low-grade to moderate-grade dysplasia, the need of extended resection is controversial (White et al. 2007; Tanaka et al. 2012; Chari et al. 2002).

To reduce operative time, we have found it useful to excise a segment of the pancreas from the end to be examined intraoperatively before we remove the entire specimen, thus giving the pathologist ample time to perform this exam. A 3–4-mm slice is enough and should be done with the scalpel rather than the cautery, to facilitate the interpretation, which can often be challenging for the pathologist. If the margin shows tumor is present, we extend the resection a few centimeters and obtain a new margin. The process is usually continued until a negative margin is obtained, potentially leading to total pancreatectomy.

12.5.3 *Intraoperative Pancreatoscopy and Intraoperative Ultrasound*

At the Massachusetts General Hospital, we have not found that intraoperative ultrasound adds much more to the preoperative imaging. However, in selected patients we use intraoperative pancreatoscopy. This allows for inspection of the ductal system of the remaining pancreas and can potentially identify "skip" lesions if they are macroscopic. The presence of these skip lesions has been proposed based on recurrence of IPMN in the remaining pancreas in the setting of a truly negative transection margin and is described in about 6–19 % of MD-IPMN (Sauvanet et al. 2010; Yelamali et al. 2012). Pancreatoscopy can be done using the laparoscopic choledochoscope, which is small enough to fit in a 4-mm pancreatic duct.

12.5.4 *Limited Anatomic and Nonanatomic Resection*

Middle (central) pancreatectomy is an alternative technique that preserves pancreatic parenchyma and reduces the risk of post-resectional endocrine and exocrine insufficiency. In a large series from the Massachusetts General Hospital and the University of Verona, about 6 % of middle pancreatectomies were performed for MD-IPMN (Crippa et al. 2007). In this series, postsurgical new-onset diabetes was only 4 % in patients undergoing middle resection vs. 27 % in those with extended distal pancreatectomy, while the pancreatic fistula rate (ISGPF B+C) was comparable (17 % vs. 13 %). For reconstruction either antecolic, end-to-side, mucosa-to-mucosa, Roux-en-Y pancreaticojejunostomy or a pancreaticogastrostomy can be made. Routinely we secure the pancreaticoenteric anastomosis with a small stent (a 5-Fr pediatric feeding tube or equivalent), which is placed in the main pancreatic duct while performing the anastomosis. Our long-term results, however, indicate that the risk of recurrence (either in the cephalic or the caudal end) is high (33 %), and therefore middle pancreatectomy is only very rarely utilized for MD-IPMN.

12.5.5 *Laparoscopic vs. Open Resection*

Since the first description of laparoscopic distal pancreatectomies two decades ago, laparoscopic distal resection of the pancreas has slowly emerged to a standardized technique (Soper et al. 1994; Gagner and Pomp 1997). Multiple series have shown that laparoscopic pancreatic resection is feasible and safe. Lower intraoperative blood loss, reduced pain and analgesic requirements, earlier return of bowel function, and shorter recovery and hospital stay have all been reported. Finally cosmetic results appear superior compared to standard incision. At the present time, approximately 27 % of distal resections are performed laparoscopically; in specialized centers the percentage is as high as 50 % (Rosales-Velderrain et al. 2012).

While some authors claim that in general oncological results are comparable between open and laparoscopic techniques, the international consensus guidelines do not comment on the laparoscopic resection of MD-IPMN. As discussed prior, achieving negative margins in MD-IPMN can necessitate stepwise extension of the resection and therefore conversion to a standard resection.

12.5.6 Preservation of the Spleen vs. Splenectomy

Splenic preservation is reasonable in all patients undergoing distal pancreatectomy for benign MD-IPMN, if the patient does not have an enlarged spleen. Preservation of the spleen can be performed with or without preservation of the splenic artery and vein. One widely used technique, where the splenic vein and artery are taken proximal and distal to the point of resection, leaving blood supply to the spleen through the short gastric vessels (i.e., the Warshaw operation), is likewise feasible in open and laparoscopic distal pancreatectomy. Preserving the spleen with this method is associated with shorter operative time and decreased blood loss and worthwhile due to the role of the spleen in the innate and adaptive immune system. . The increased flow via these collaterals results in vascular dilation (Ferrone et al. 2011; Warshaw 1988). Several series confirmed the safety of this technique with very low postoperative failure rate of 1.9 %. Even though this approach results in perigastric varices, which are radiologically identified in 25 % of patients (Ferrone et al. 2011), no bleeding complications have been described during long-time follow-up.

References

Aso T, Ohtsuka T, Ideno N, Kono H, Nagayoshi Y, Mori Y, et al. Diagnostic significance of a dilated orifice of the duodenal papilla in intraductal papillary mucinous neoplasm of the pancreas. Gastrointest Endosc. 2012;76(2):313–20. doi:10.1016/j.gie.2012.03.682.

Chari ST, Yadav D, Smyrk TC, DiMagno EP, Miller LJ, Raimondo M, et al. Study of recurrence after surgical resection of intraductal papillary mucinous neoplasm of the pancreas. Gastroenterology. 2002;123(5):1500–7.

Couvelard A, Sauvanet A, Kianmanesh R, Hammel P, Colnot N, Levy P, et al. Frozen sectioning of the pancreatic cut surface during resection of intraductal papillary mucinous neoplasms of the pancreas is useful and reliable: a prospective evaluation. Ann Surg. 2005;242(6):774–8. discussion 778–780.

Crippa S, Bassi C, Warshaw AL, Falconi M, Partelli S, Thayer SP, et al. Middle pancreatectomy: indications, short- and long-term operative outcomes. Ann Surg. 2007;246(1):69–76. doi:10.1097/01.sla.0000262790.51512.57.

Crippa S, Fernandez-Del Castillo C, Salvia R, Finkelstein D, Bassi C, Dominguez I, et al. Mucin-producing neoplasms of the pancreas: an analysis of distinguishing clinical and epidemiologic characteristics. Clin Gastroenterol Hepatol. 2010;8(2):213–9. doi:10.1016/j.cgh.2009.10.001.

Fernandez-Del Castillo C, Adsay NV. Intraductal papillary mucinous neoplasms of the pancreas. Gastroenterology. 2010;139(3):708–13. doi:10.1053/j.gastro.2010.07.025. 713.e701-702.

Ferrone CR, Konstantinidis IT, Sahani DV, Wargo JA, Fernandez-del Castillo C, Warshaw AL. Twenty-three years of the Warshaw operation for distal pancreatectomy with preservation of the spleen. Ann Surg. 2011;253(6):1136–9. doi:10.1097/SLA.0b013e318212c1e2.

Gagner M, Pomp A. Laparoscopic pancreatic resection: is it worthwhile? J Gastrointest Surg. 1997;1(1):20–5. discussion 25–26.

Manfredi R, Graziani R, Motton M, Mantovani W, Baltieri S, Tognolini A, et al. Main pancreatic duct intraductal papillary mucinous neoplasms: accuracy of MR imaging in differentiation between benign and malignant tumors compared with histopathologic analysis. Radiology. 2009;253(1):106–15. doi:10.1148/radiol.2531080604.

Ohno E, Hirooka Y, Itoh A, Ishigami M, Katano Y, Ohmiya N, et al. Intraductal papillary mucinous neoplasms of the pancreas: differentiation of malignant and benign tumors by endoscopic ultrasonography findings of mural nodules. Ann Surg. 2011. doi:10.1097/SLA.0b013e31819edle5.

Rosales-Velderrain A, Bowers SP, Goldberg RF, Clarke TM, Buchanan MA, Stauffer JA, et al. National trends in resection of the distal pancreas. World J Gastroenterol WJG. 2012;18(32):4342–9. doi:10.3748/wjg.v18.i32.4342.

Salvia R, Fernandez-Del Castillo C, Bassi C, Thayer SP, Falconi M, Mantovani W, et al. Main-duct intraductal papillary mucinous neoplasms of the pancreas: clinical predictors of malignancy and long-term survival following resection. Ann Surg. 2004;239(5):678–85. discussion 685–677.

Salvia R, Crippa S, Partelli S, Armatura G, Malleo G, Paini M, et al. Differences between main-duct and branch-duct intraductal papillary mucinous neoplasms of the pancreas. World J Gastrointest Surg. 2010;2(10):342–6. doi:10.4240/wjgs.v2.i10.342.

Sauvanet A, Couvelard A, Belghiti J. Role of frozen section assessment for intraductal papillary and mucinous tumor of the pancreas. World J Gastrointest Surg. 2010;2(10):352–8. doi:10.4240/wjgs.v2.i10.352.

Soper NJ, Brunt LM, Dunnegan DL, Meininger TA. Laparoscopic distal pancreatectomy in the porcine model. Surg Endosc. 1994;8(1):57–60. discussion 60–51.

Sugiyama M, Izumisato Y, Abe N, Masaki T, Mori T, Atomi Y. Predictive factors for malignancy in intraductal papillary-mucinous tumours of the pancreas. Br J Surg. 2003;90(10):1244–9. doi:10.1002/bjs.4265.

Suzuki Y, Atomi Y, Sugiyama M, Isaji S, Inui K, Kimura W, et al. Cystic neoplasm of the pancreas: a Japanese multiinstitutional study of intraductal papillary mucinous tumor and mucinous cystic tumor. Pancreas. 2004;28(3):241–6.

Takuma K, Kamisawa T, Anjiki H, Egawa N, Kurata M, Honda G, et al. Predictors of malignancy and natural history of main-duct intraductal papillary mucinous neoplasms of the pancreas. Pancreas. 2011;40(3):371–5. doi:10.1097/MPA.0b013e3182056a83.

Tanaka M, Chari S, Adsay V, Fernandez-Del Castillo C, Falconi M, Shimizu M, et al. International consensus guidelines for management of intraductal papillary mucinous neoplasms and mucinous cystic neoplasms of the pancreas. Pancreatology. 2006;6:17–32. doi:10.1159/000090023.

Tanaka M, Fernandez-Del Castillo C, Adsay V, Chari S, Falconi M, Jang J-Y, et al. International consensus guidelines 2012 for the management of IPMN and MCN of the pancreas. Pancreatology. 2012;12(3):183–97. doi:10.1016/j.pan.2012.04.004.

Uehara H, Ishikawa O, Ikezawa K, Kawada N, Inoue T, Takakura R, et al. A natural course of main duct intraductal papillary mucinous neoplasm of the pancreas with lower likelihood of malignancy. Pancreas. 2010;39(5):653–7. doi:10.1097/MPA.0b013e3181c81b52.

Warshaw AL. Conservation of the spleen with distal pancreatectomy. Arch Surg. 1988;123(5):550–3.

White R, D'Angelica M, Katabi N, Tang L, Klimstra D, Fong Y, et al. Fate of the remnant pancreas after resection of noninvasive intraductal papillary mucinous neoplasm. J Am Coll Surg. 2007;204(5):987–93. doi:10.1016/j.jamcollsurg.2006.12.040. discussion 993–985.

Yelamali A, Mansard MJ, Dama R, Rebela P, Rao GV, Reddy DN. Intraoperative pancreatoscopy with narrow band imaging: a novel method for assessment of resection margins in case of intraductal papillary mucinous neoplasm. Surg Endosc. 2012. doi:10.1007/s00464-012-2365-6.

Chapter 13
Method of Resection of Branch-Duct IPMN

Anne Marie Lennon and Christopher L. Wolfgang

Abstract IPMNs of the pancreas are precursor lesions to pancreatic ductal adenocarcinoma. The risk of malignancy in IPMN is based on further subclassification into three types: main-duct IPMN (MD-IPMN), branch-duct IPMN (BD-IPMN), and mixed-type IPMN (MT-IPMN). The malignant potential of MD and MT is substantial and most should undergo resection. The BD-IPMN subtype is more indolent and the decision to resect is more selective. The international consensus guidelines for the management of cystic neoplasms known as the "Sendai criteria" or "Tanaka criteria" provide recommendations for the management of BD-IPMN based on risk of malignancy. Indications for resection of BD-IPMN include the high-risk stigmata of jaundice and the presence of a solid component. Since the decision to resect IPMN is based on concern for malignancy, a formal oncological operation should be performed. The outcome of resected benign BD-IPMN is good. However, the risk of progressive or new IPMN disease, including invasive cancer, in patients undergoing resection of BD-IPMN is significant, and these individuals need to be followed closely and indefinitely.

Keywords Branch-duct IPMN (BD-IPMN) • Indications for surgery • International consensus guidelines • Invasive IPMN • Management • Pancreatic ductal adenocarcinoma • Sendai criteria • Tanaka criteria

13.1 Introduction

The surgical management of IPMN depends on the risk of malignancy and this is based on the classification of these lesions into three subtypes. These include main-duct IPMN (MD-IPMN), branch-duct IPMN (BD-IPMN), and mixed-type IPMN

Disclosures: Neither author has any disclosures.

A.M. Lennon • C.L. Wolfgang (✉)
The Johns Hopkins Hospital, Baltimore, MD, USA
e-mail: cwolfga2@jhmi.edu

M. Tanaka (ed.), *Intraductal Papillary Mucinous Neoplasm of the Pancreas*,
DOI 10.1007/978-4-431-54472-2_13, © Springer Japan 2014

(MT-IPMN). MD-IPMN is defined as having segmental or diffuse dilation of the main pancreatic duct to ≥5 mm in the absence of a dominant cyst. BD-IPMN is defined as an IPMN with at least one cyst measuring >5 mm in diameter in the presence of a normal or minimally dilated pancreatic duct. A mixed-type IPMN has both one or more dominant cysts and a pancreatic duct measuring >5 mm. The risk of malignancy is relatively high in both MD-IPMN and MT-IPMN (Tanaka et al. 2006). In one large retrospective series of resected patients, the rate of invasive cancer in MD-IPMN was 44 % and in MT-IPMN was 45 %. Moreover, MD-IPMN and MT-IPMN are associated with high-grade dysplasia in 62.2 % and 57.6 % of resected patients, respectively (Tanaka et al. 2012). BD-IPMN is a more indolent subtype of IPMN and associated with a lower risk of malignancy. In contrast, BD-IPMN has a much lower risk of malignant transformation, with an annual rate of 2–3 % (Kang et al. 2011; Levy et al. 2006). Therefore, the algorithm for the management of BD-IPMN differs from that of MD- or MT-IPMN. The goal of this chapter is to define the indications and type of resection performed for BD-IPMN. Resection of MD-IPMN and MT-IPMN is discussed elsewhere.

The most important aspect to the optimal management of BD-IPMN is differentiating patients who will benefit by resection from those who can safely undergo observation. IPMN undergoes a spectrum of dysplastic changes that range from low-grade dysplasia to high-grade and finally invasive carcinoma. Although it is unclear based on available literature, it is generally believed that patients with low- or intermediate-grade dysplasia do not benefit from surgical resection. On the other hand, it is generally felt that patients with high-grade dysplasia will more likely progress to invasive cancer and should undergo resection. The outcome following resection of IPMN with high-grade dysplasia is good. The 5-year survival in patients with resected IPMN found to have high-grade dysplasia is reported at 93.3 % (Hwang et al. 2012) to 100 % (Salvia et al. 2004). Once IPMN progresses to invasive cancer, the survival rate falls significantly with rates ranging between 31 % and 62.1 % (Hwang et al. 2012; Salvia et al. 2004; Sohn et al. 2004; Suzuki et al. 2004; Nagai et al. 2008). Clearly patients with localized IPMN-associated PDAC should undergo resection and have the potential for a cure. However, the optimal situation would be to identify and resect patients who have an IPMN that harbors high-grade dysplasia. In this group surgery alone is essentially curative and the risk of operation is justified by the presumed benefit of cancer prevention. Unfortunately, no preoperative indicators that differentiate high-grade dysplasia from lower grades exist. The current imaging modalities are able to differentiate among the three subtypes of IPMN with relatively good reliability but are poor for predicting dysplasia (Tanaka et al. 2012). The addition of cyst fluid analysis obtained by endoscopic ultrasound (EUS) adds little to the ability to identify high-grade lesions. The level of cyst fluid CEA does not correlate with degree of dysplasia (van der Waaij et al. 2005; Frossard et al. 2003; Khalid et al. 2009; Sreenarasimhaiah et al. 2009; Shen et al. 2009; Sawhney et al. 2009) and cytology is often hard to interpret. Moreover, the rate of false-positive and false-negative for classification of grade is significant (van der Waaij et al. 2005; Frossard et al. 2003; Khalid et al. 2009; Sreenarasimhaiah et al. 2009; Shen et al. 2009; Sawhney et al. 2009). The current imaging modalities are relatively good as regards identifying invasive cancer associated with BD-IPMN. Imaging features associated with invasive cancer include significant dilatation of the main pancreatic and common bile ducts, an abrupt cutoff and associated mass in a dilated duct, a solid component within a cyst, or a solid mass in a gland with associated cysts (Sahani et al. 2005). As a result of the inability to differentiate among the degrees of dysplasia along with the ability to reliably identify cancer, the current guidelines are designed to identify patients with an IPMN malignancy (invasive cancer) and not high-grade precursor lesions.

13.2 Management Algorithm for BD-IPMN

In 2006, a group of experts convened in Sendai at the International Association of Pancreatology and created a set of guidelines for the management of cystic pancreatic neoplasms (Tanaka et al. 2006). These recommendations are known as the "Sendai criteria" or the "Tanaka criteria" and are based on the available literature at that time which mainly consisted of retrospective series. These guidelines are safe when appropriately applied and function well in stratifying patients for observation or resection (Nagai et al. 2008). Recommendations continue to undergo revision and validation due to the challenge of diagnosis and incomplete understanding of malignant transformation of these cysts. An updated version of these guidelines was published in 2012 (Tanaka et al. 2012). The revised criteria serve to clarify the definition, management, and surveillance protocol of IPMNs. In the 2012 version, IPMNs with significant imaging findings or clinical parameters are classified as having either "high-risk stigmata" or "worrisome features" based on the concern for invasive cancer. "High-risk stigmata" of malignancy in BD-IPMN is defined as (1) obstructive jaundice in a patient with a cystic lesion of the head of the pancreas or (2) enhancing solid component within a cyst (mural nodule). Patients with BD-IPMN who are found to have high-risk stigmata of malignancy should undergo a resection.

In BD-IPMNs without "high-risk stigmata," an assessment should be made for "worrisome features" including (1) pancreatitis, (2) cyst ≥3 cm, (3) thickened or enhancing cyst walls, (4) non-enhancing mural nodule, and (5) abrupt change in caliber of pancreatic duct with distal atrophy. Those IPMNs with "worrisome features" should undergo EUS evaluation with evaluation of cyst fluid. If EUS identifies a definite mural nodule, suspicious features, or cytological atypia, then surgery should be considered. Otherwise, follow-up with EUS or cross-sectional imaging is recommended with timing based on cyst size.

The accuracy and safety of the consensus guidelines have been studied. The sensitivity in identifying malignancy was determined in a single-institution retrospective study that reviewed 84 patients with BD-IPMN who underwent resection over a 22-year period (Nagai et al. 2008). Sixty-nine patients had one or more indications for resection by the original international consensus criteria. Thirty-six of thirty-seven patients with malignancy had indications. The authors concluded that the sensitivity for predicting malignancy was 97 % (Sadakari et al. 2010). In addition, a large bi-institutional study from Massachusetts General Hospital and the University of Verona identified 145 patients who underwent resection with pathologically confirmed BD-IPMN (Rodriguez et al. 2007). Their analysis revealed that all neoplasms with cancer were detected by the original consensus criteria.

In contrast, recent work also from the Massachusetts General Hospital suggests that there may be insufficient diagnostic accuracy with current imaging to formulate appropriate treatment strategies (Correa-Gallego et al. 2010). In this retrospective study of 330 patients with incidentally identified cystic pancreatic lesions, preoperative and final histologic diagnosis were correlated in the 136 (41 %) patients undergoing resection. The authors found that although most lesions preoperatively identified as MD-IPMNs or serous cystadenomas were confirmed after resection, BD-IPMN and mucinous cystic neoplasms were less accurately diagnosed, with only 64 % and 60 % accuracy, respectively. Of particular concern was the finding that 20 % of specimens with a BD-IPMN diagnosis on imaging demonstrated main-duct involvement thus conveying a worse prognosis and need for surgical resection. The authors conclude that better diagnostic methods will be necessary to formulate treatment strategies.

13.3 Extent of Operation

The goal for resection of BD-IPMN is either the prevention of cancer or removal of a localized cancer depending on the circumstance. In either case, basic principles of an oncological resection of pancreatic malignancy should apply. This includes removal of the primary lesion with an adequate margin of normal tissue and a regional lymphadenectomy. Thus, the operations employed should include pancreaticoduodenectomy for lesions of the head, neck, and uncinate and a distal pancreatectomy for lesions of the body and tail. Occasionally, a central pancreatectomy may be appropriate. The rationale behind a formal resection for even benign disease in BD-IPMN is that the methods to preoperatively differentiate benign from malignant are imprecise. Thus, prior to operation in a patient who meets the consensus criteria for resection, the presence of malignancy is not known but presumed to be high.

An interesting feature of IPMN that is an important consideration in surgical management is the high rate of multifocal disease. BD-IPMNs have been reported to be multifocal in up to 30 % of cases (Wu et al. 2011) and are felt by some to be a field defect in which the entire pancreas is at risk. Currently, resection of BD-IPMN is geared at removal of the predominant lesion, and at times a clinically apparent IPMN may intentionally be left behind to preserve pancreatic parenchyma. This practice appropriately balances the detrimental long-term effects of both endocrine and exocrine insufficiency with an acceptable reduction in risk of malignancy. It must be noted however that the potential of developing progressive IPMN disease or even IPMN malignancy following resection of a benign IPMN is significant

(He et al. 2013). As described in more detail below, following resection of a benign IPMN, patients continue to need surveillance of their pancreatic remnant.

While complete resection through pancreaticoduodenectomy or distal pancreatectomy has been utilized by most centers, a multi-institutional international series from Indiana University and Institut Paoli-Calmettes (France) evaluated the use of enucleation for side-branch IPMNs (Turrini et al. 2011). They reviewed 107 patients undergoing pancreatic surgery for BD-IPMN of the pancreatic head/uncinate—7 undergoing enucleation and 100 undergoing pancreaticoduodenectomy. They found that the enucleation group had a significantly shorter operative time and lower blood loss and a non-statistically significantly higher fistula rate. Despite this, based on oncological principles, enucleation of BD-IPMN is not an adequate resection.

13.4 Follow-Up After Resection

A growing body of evidence suggests that a resection of a benign BD-IPMN reduces but does not eliminate the risk of developing pancreatic cancer (He et al. 2013; Moriya and Traverso 2012; Miller et al. 2011; Cauley et al. 2012; Chari et al. 2002; White et al. 2007). Following resection of a benign IPMN, several investigators report the development of subsequent BD-IPMN or progression of an existing BD-IPMN in up to 20 % of patients. Moreover, numerous reports now exist in which pancreatic cancer developed in patients who underwent resection of benign IPMN in a remote location (He et al. 2013; Miller et al. 2011). Factors that predict subsequent clinically significant IPMN are not well characterized. The Johns Hopkins group reported that family history of pancreatic cancer is an independent risk factor for subsequent disease (He et al. 2013). Moreover, the work of this group suggests that the finding of high-grade dysplasia in the primary lesion is a marker for relatively aggressive biology since this was found in all patients who subsequently developed a cancer. Based on this recent work, it is clear that just as patients with newly diagnosed BD-IPMN need at least close follow-up, so do those who have undergone resection of BD-IPMN. Close attention should be paid to those who undergo resection of high-grade dysplasia. In general, patients with cysts in the remnant pancreas should be followed as per BD-IPMN protocol. Those without cysts can undergo surveillance yearly.

13.5 Summary

The management of BD-IPMN is based on the risk of malignancy. Those patients who have low-malignant potential lesions can undergo careful surveillance, while those with high-risk stigmata should undergo an oncological resection. Outcomes of resected benign BD-IPMN are good. Long-term follow-up is necessary even in patients undergoing resection of benign IPMN.

References

Cauley CE, Waters JA, Dumas RP, et al. Outcomes of primary surveillance for intraductal papillary mucinous neoplasm. J Gastrointest Surg. 2012;16(2):258–67. discussion 266.

Chari ST, Yadav D, Smyrk TC, et al. Study of recurrence after surgical resection of intraductal papillary mucinous neoplasm of the pancreas. Gastroenterology. 2002;123(5):1500–7.

Correa-Gallego C et al. Incidental pancreatic cysts: do we really know what we are watching? Pancreatology. 2010;10(2–3):144–50.

Frossard JL, Amouyal P, Amouyal G, et al. Performance of endosonography-guided fine needle aspiration and biopsy in the diagnosis of pancreatic cystic lesions. Am J Gastroenterol. 2003;98:1516–24.

He J, Cameron JL, Ahuja N, Makary MA, Hirose K, Choti MA, et al. Is it necessary to follow patients after resection of a benign pancreatic intraductal papillary mucinous neoplasm? J Am Coll Surg. 2013;216(4):657–65.

Hwang DW, Jang JY, Lee SE, et al. Clinicopathologic analysis of surgically proven intraductal papillary mucinous neoplasms of the pancreas in SNUH: a 15-year experience at a single academic institution. Langenbecks Arch Surg. 2012;397:93–102.

Kang MJ, Jang JY, Kim SJ, et al. Cyst growth rate predicts malignancy in patients with branch duct intraductal papillary mucinous neoplasms. Clin Gastroenterol Hepatol. 2011;9:87–93.

Khalid A, Zahid M, Finkelstein SD, et al. Pancreatic cyst fluid DNA analysis in evaluating pancreatic cysts: a report of the PANDA study. Gastrointest Endosc. 2009;69:1095–102.

Levy P, Jouannaud V, O'Toole D, et al. Natural history of intraductal papillary mucinous tumors of the pancreas: actuarial risk of malignancy. Clin Gastroenterol Hepatol. 2006;4:460–8.

Miller JR, Meyer JE, Waters JA, et al. Outcome of the pancreatic remnant following segmental pancreatectomy for non-invasive intraductal papillary mucinous neoplasm. HPB (Oxford). 2011;13(11):759–66.

Moriya T, Traverso W. Fate of the pancreatic remnant after resection for an intraductal papillary mucinous neoplasm: a longitudinal level II cohort study. Arch Surg. 2012;147(6):528–34.

Nagai K, Doi R, Kida A, et al. Intraductal papillary mucinous neoplasms of the pancreas: clinicopathologic characteristics and long-term follow-up after resection. World J Surg. 2008;32:271–8. discussion 279–80.

Rodriguez JR et al. Branch-duct intraductal papillary mucinous neoplasms: observations in 145 patients who underwent resection. Gastroenterology. 2007;133(1):72–9. quiz 309–10.

Sadakari Y et al. Cyst size indicates malignant transformation in branch duct intraductal papillary mucinous neoplasm of the pancreas without mural nodules. Pancreas. 2010;39(2):232–6.

Sahani DV, Kadavigere R, Saokar A, et al. Cystic pancreatic lesions: a simple imaging-based classification system for guiding management. Radiographics. 2005;25:1471–84.

Salvia R, Fernandez-del Castillo C, Bassi C, et al. Main-duct intraductal papillary mucinous neoplasms of the pancreas: clinical predictors of malignancy and long-term survival following resection. Ann Surg. 2004;239:678–85. discussion 685–7.

Sawhney MS, Devarajan S, O'Farrel P, et al. Comparison of carcinoembryonic antigen and molecular analysis in pancreatic cyst fluid. Gastrointest Endosc. 2009;69:1106–10.

Shen J, Brugge WR, Dimaio CJ, et al. Molecular analysis of pancreatic cyst fluid: a comparative analysis with current practice of diagnosis. Cancer. 2009;117:217–27.

Sohn TA, Yeo CJ, Cameron JL, et al. Intraductal papillary mucinous neoplasms of the pancreas: an updated experience. Ann Surg. 2004;239:788–97. discussion 797–9.

Sreenarasimhaiah J, Lara LF, Jazrawi SF, et al. A comparative analysis of pancreas cyst fluid CEA and histology with DNA mutational analysis in the detection of mucin producing or malignant cysts. JOP. 2009;10:163–8.

Suzuki Y, Atomi Y, Sugiyama M, et al. Cystic neoplasm of the pancreas: a Japanese multiinstitutional study of intraductal papillary mucinous tumor and mucinous cystic tumor. Pancreas. 2004;28:241–6.

Tanaka M et al. International consensus guidelines for management of intraductal papillary mucinous neoplasms and mucinous cystic neoplasms of the pancreas. Pancreatology. 2006;6(1–2):17–32.

Tanaka M, Fernandez-Del Castillo C, Adsay V, et al. International consensus guidelines 2012 for the management of IPMN and MCN of the pancreas. Pancreatology. 2012;12:183–97.

Turrini O et al. Side-branch intraductal papillary mucinous neoplasms of the pancreatic head/uncinate: resection or enucleation? HPB (Oxford). 2011;13(2):126–31.

van der Waaij LA, van Dullemen HM, Porte RJ. Cyst fluid analysis in the differential diagnosis of pancreatic cystic lesions: a pooled analysis. Gastrointest Endosc. 2005;62:383–9.

White R, D'Angelica M, Katabi N, et al. Fate of the remnant pancreas after resection of noninvasive intraductal papillary mucinous neoplasm. J Am Coll Surg. 2007;204(5):987–93. discussion 993–985.

Wu J, Matthaei H, Maitra A, et al. Recurrent GNAS mutations define an unexpected pathway for pancreatic cyst development. Sci Transl Med. 2011;3:92ra66.

Chapter 14
Timing of Resection of Branch Duct IPMN

Jin-Young Jang

Abstract Branch duct intraductal papillary mucinous neoplasms (IPMNs) carry a moderate risk of malignancy, making resection a possible treatment. However, the annual risk of malignancy is only 2–3 % per year and these slow-growing lesions occur mainly in males during their seventh decade of life, who have relatively short life expectancy. Moreover, since surgery is accompanied by a relatively high morbidity rate and function loss, resection may not be indicated in some patients. Factors found to predict the risk of malignancy include size >3 cm; the presence of mural nodules, main duct dilatation (>5 mm), and cyst wall thickening; growth rate, cytology (+), and the presence of tumor markers. Factors that should be considered in deciding whether to perform surgery include age and life expectancy, whether the general condition of the patient is sufficient for major surgery, patient desire for cure, and tumor location. The complexity of making decisions in regard to patients with BD-IPMN has precluded the development of standard treatment guidelines applicable to every patient. Rather, treatment must be tailored to the clinical situations of individual patients.

Keywords Branch duct • Consensus guideline • Indication of surgery • Intraductal papillary mucinous neoplasm • Malignancy predicting factor

14.1 Introduction

Intraductal papillary mucinous neoplasms (IPMNs) of the main pancreatic duct are tumors characterized by dilatation of the main pancreatic duct and secretion of mucin. IPMNs involving the main pancreatic duct have a relatively high risk

J.-Y. Jang (✉)
Department of Surgery, Seoul National University College of Medicine,
28 Yongon-dong, Chongno-gu, Seoul 110-744, South Korea
e-mail: jangjy4@snu.ac.kr

M. Tanaka (ed.), *Intraductal Papillary Mucinous Neoplasm of the Pancreas*,
DOI 10.1007/978-4-431-54472-2_14, © Springer Japan 2014

(36–100 %) of progression to malignancy and invasive carcinoma. The clinical and pathological characteristics of these tumors have been described, and treatment guidelines have been developed, including surgical resection of tumor involving the main pancreatic duct (Longnecker et al. 2005; Tanaka et al. 2006, 2012).

In contrast, branch duct (BD)-type IPMNs have a lower risk of malignancy (6.3–46.5 %), raising questions about the necessity of surgical resection and the timing of the operation (Tanaka et al. 2012; Jang et al. 2008; Hwang et al. 2011). The annual risk of malignancy is only 2–3 % per year and these slow-growing lesions occur mainly in males during their seventh decade of life, who have relatively short life expectancy. Moreover, since surgery is accompanied by a relatively high morbidity rate and function loss, resection may not be indicated (Kang et al. 2011; Lévy et al. 2006). Observation alone may be appropriate in selected patients without the factors that predict malignancy. Determining appropriate patient management, including the timing of surgery, should be based on the natural history of BD-IPMNs, the presence of factors predicting malignancy, each patient's general condition and willingness to undergo surgery, lesion location, and the presence of symptoms.

In this chapter, we will discuss the clinical factors determining the optimal timing of surgery in patients with BD-IPMN.

14.2 Considered Factors for Surgery

14.2.1 Risk Factors for Malignancy

Recent consensus guidelines have described malignancy-related factors as "worrisome features" and "high-risk stigmata" (Tanaka et al. 2012). "Worrisome features" included cysts ≥3 cm in diameter, thickened cyst walls, non-enhanced mural nodules, MPD size 5–9 mm, an abrupt change in MPD caliber with distal pancreatic atrophy, and lymphadenopathy. "High-risk stigmata" included MPD >10 mm and an enhanced solid component. Due to the lack of international standards for cyst size, diameter of the dilated main duct, and imaging methods used to measure risk factors, the clinical importance of each factor is difficult to determine, even after meta-analysis (Anand et al. 2013).

14.2.1.1 Size

The risk of malignancy and size criteria for BD-IPMN have been found to vary, depending on the characteristics of the patients enrolled. At the extremes are some groups that advocate observation alone, regardless of tumor size, and those that indicate that surgical resection be considered for all patients with BD-IPMN based on the high risk of malignancy of even small-sized BD-IPMNs (Salvia et al. 2007; Arlix et al. 2012; Fritz et al. 2012). Others, however, have found that a size of 2–4 cm can predict malignancy (Jang et al. 2008; Shimizu et al. 2013; Nagai et al. 2009).

Size>3cm Meta-Analysis

Study Name	Odds ratio	Lower limit	Upper limit	Z-Value	p-Value
Nagai	27.413	10.643	70.608	6.859	0.000
schmidt	472.235	142.929	1560.261	10.098	0.000
Rodriguez	44.600	19.837	100.274	9.187	0.000
Terris	6668.333	215.417	206421.284	5.028	0.000
Kang	22.344	5.207	95.892	4.180	0.000
Tang	62.750	6.300	625.053	3.529	0.000
Carbognin	29.726	1.468	602.119	2.210	0.027
Fukushima	63.413	2.845	1413.557	2.620	0.009
Sugiyama	499.500	41.048	6078.213	4.874	0.000
wakabayashi	15.822	0.826	303.057	1.833	0.067
Maguchi	146.255	34.577	618.623	6.775	0.000
Sadakari	3.727	0.207	67.243	0.891	0.373
ohtsuka	6.903	1.973	24.147	3.024	0.002
akita	55.833	13.434	232.043	5.534	0.000
woo sm	75.337	23.939	237.094	7.389	0.000
Takeshita	172.114	34.325	863.027	6.258	0.000
	62.391	30.830	126.262	11.492	0.000

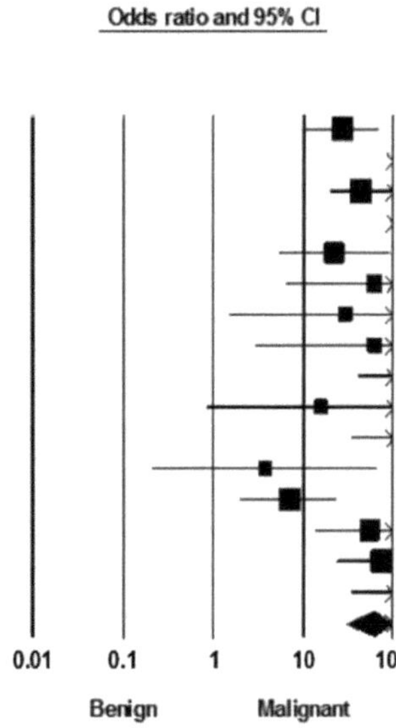

Fig. 14.1 Forest plot for cyst size >3 cm and risk of malignancy. Sixteen studies were included: pooled OR 62.4 [95 % CI 30.8, 126.3] (Anand et al. 2013)

The development of imaging techniques has shown that radiological characteristics, such as mural nodule size and cyst wall thickening, are more important indicators of malignancy than cyst size itself. However, cyst size remains a useful criterion, because of its ease of measurement and greater uniformity than other radiological parameters.

A recent meta-analysis found that cyst size >3 cm was associated with a substantially increased risk of malignancy (pooled odds ratio [OR] 62.4, 95 % confidence interval [CI] 30.8, 126.3) and that this criterion was most strongly associated with malignant IPMN (Fig. 14.1) (Anand et al. 2013). Thus, cyst size may play a major role in deciding whether to surgically resect BD-IPMNs.

14.2.1.2 Mural Nodule

The presence or absence of mural nodules is important in determining whether to perform surgery to remove IPMNs. One study found that 19 of 23 patients (83 %) with mural nodules in an IPMN had a diagnosis of malignancy (Rodriguez et al. 2007). Other smaller studies also indicated that approximately 80 % of IPMNs with mural nodules are carcinomas (Akita et al. 2011; Yamashita et al. 2013).

It is sometimes difficult, however, to precisely evaluate whether mural nodules are present. In particular, distinguishing mural nodules from mucous clots is difficult using either multidetector computed tomography (CT) or endoscopic sonography (Zhong et al. 2012; Yamashita et al. 2013; Uehara et al. 2011).

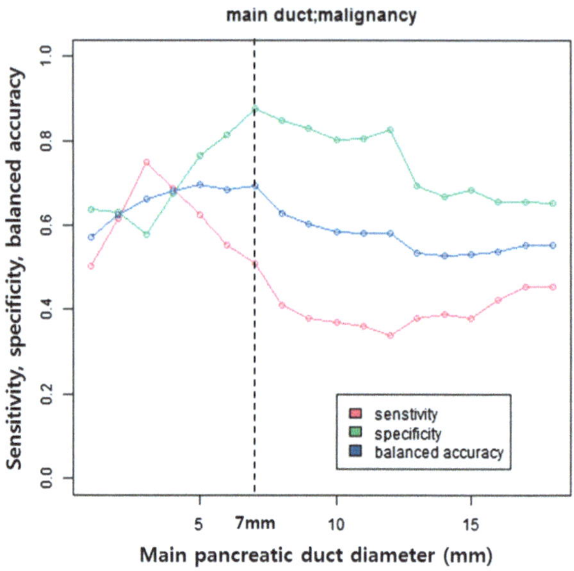

Fig. 14.2 Sensitivity and specificity of malignancy prediction at the main duct diameter of 7 mm with a malignancy prediction probability of 0.3 was 51.1 % and 87.6 %

Despite the heterogeneity of diagnostic tools and the definitions of mural nodules, the presence of a mural nodule within the cyst is a strong risk factor for malignancy (OR 9.3, 95 % CI 5.3, 16.1) (Anand et al. 2013).

14.2.1.3 Combined Main Duct Dilatation

IPMNs are difficult to classify, since no definitive standards have been developed to distinguish among main duct type, mixed type, and branch duct type. Many patients with BD-IPMN show marked dilatation of the main pancreatic duct, making these lesions main- or mixed-type IPMN. Although there may be discrepancy (20–30 %) between pathologic tumor involvement in the main duct and main duct dilatation itself, combined main duct dilatation was found to increase the risk of malignancy in patients with BD-IPMN. Previous IAP guidelines indicated that dilatation of 10 mm was a criterion for main duct IPMN, whereas the new IAP guidelines have broadened this criterion, defining 6–10 mm main duct dilatation as a "worrisome feature" (Tanaka et al. 2006, 2012).

Meta-analysis has shown that a >6 mm dilatation of the main pancreatic duct was associated with an increased risk of malignancy (pooled OR 7.27, 95 % CI 3.0, 17.4) (Anand et al. 2013).

Our unpublished data on 350 patients with BD-IPMN showed that a main pancreatic duct size of 7 mm is a significant cutoff predicting malignancy. The risk of malignancy in BD-IPMN patients with combined main duct dilatation over 7 mm was comparable to that of patients with main duct IPMN (Fig. 14.2). We recommend that patients with branch duct cystic dilatation with main duct dilatation over 7 mm be diagnosed as having mixed-type or predominantly main duct-type IPMN, not BD-IPMN. Except in patients with mixed-type IPMN, we found that the risk of malignancy in patients with BD-IPMN increased in proportion to dilatation of the main duct, especially over 5 mm.

14.2.1.4 Tumor Markers

Serum concentrations of the tumor-associated glycoproteins carbohydrate antigen (CA) 19-9 and carcinoembryonic antigen (CEA) are increased in approximately 50–85 % of patients with pancreatic ductal adenocarcinoma (PDAC) (Ferrone et al. 2006). Similarly, these markers may be predictive of malignancy in patients with BD-IPMN. Although direct measurements of tumor markers in cystic fluid have been reported to predict malignancy, puncture of the cyst or p-duct cannulation is an invasive procedure, as well as carrying a risk of tumor spillage through the peritoneal cavity. Therefore, cyst puncture or p-duct cannulation is not recommended as a routine diagnostic tool in these patients (Fig. 14.3).

Measuring tumor marker concentrations in using serum or plasma is the most widely used method for most of cancer detection. For example, 74 % of patients with an invasive IPMN had increased CA19-9 concentrations, compared with only 14 % of patients with noninvasive tumors (Fritz et al. 2011). Using a cutoff level of 37 unit/mL, CA19-9 had a specificity of 85.9 %, a negative predictive value of 85.9 %, a positive predictive value of 74.0 %, and an accuracy of 81.7 % in predicting malignancy. Overall, increased serum concentrations of CA19-9 and/or CEA have been observed in 80 % of patients with an invasive IPMN but in only 18 % of patients with a noninvasive tumor ($P<0.001$). Although more evidence is needed to establish the clinical efficacy of tumor markers for the detection of malignant IPMN, noninvasive markers may be helpful in differentiating between malignant and benign IPMNs and will be an important topic for future research (Hirono et al. 2012).

14.2.1.5 Other Risk Factors

Improvements in imaging modalities have yielded finer images with markedly improved resolution. Thus, more sophisticated findings are considered predictors of malignancy, such as cyst wall thickening or enhancement and abrupt changes in the caliber of the pancreatic duct with pancreatic atrophy (Chiu et al. 2006). In addition, pancreatic cyst growth rate may predict malignancy (Rautou et al. 2008; Kang et al. 2011). Our group found that cysts that grew >2 mm/year had a significantly higher 5-year risk of malignancy than cysts that grew more slowly (45.5 % vs 1.8 %; $P<0.001$) (Kang et al. 2011). EUS-based classifications of tumor morphology have also been used to predict malignancy (Ohno et al. 2012).

Preoperative cytology may also be diagnostic in these patients (Genevay et al. 2011). Although cytology had a high positive predictive value and a high specificity,

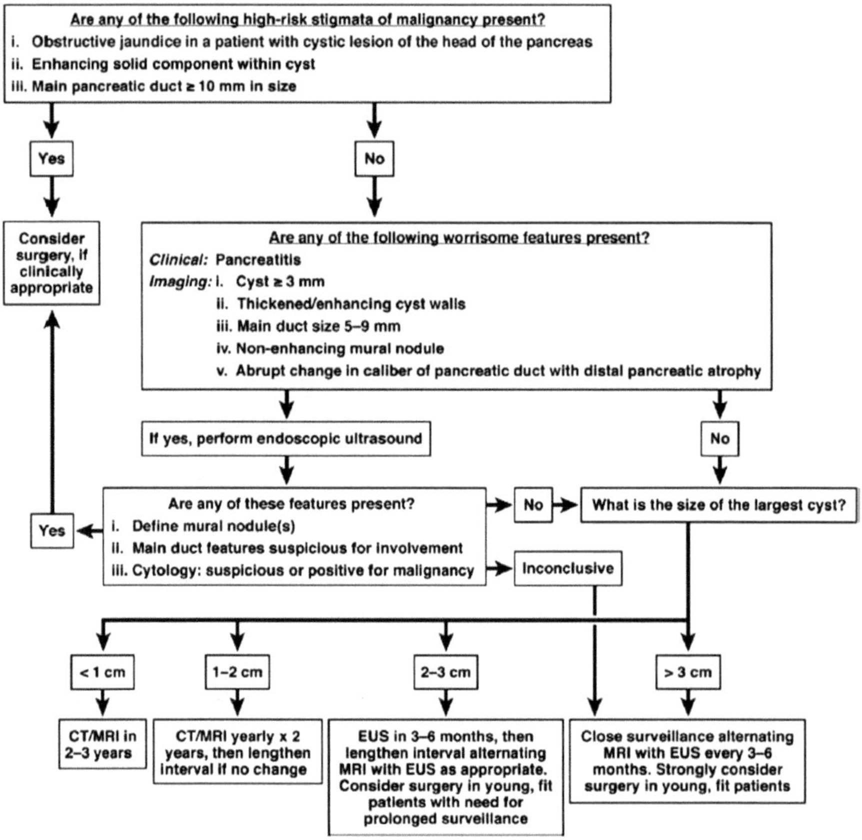

Fig. 14.3 New consensus guideline for managing patients with BD-IPMN (Tanaka et al. 2012)

it carries a risk of cyst rupture and tumor spillage due to direct puncture of the cyst. Moreover, cytology was found to have a low sensitivity and show diagnostic discrepancies (Imaoka et al. 2006).

14.2.2 Other Factors for Selecting Treatment Method

14.2.2.1 Natural History

The natural history of BD-IPMN has been found to vary widely. Since these tumors were described only recently, investigations of more patients are required to determine the natural course of BD-IPMNs in general. The annual risk of BD-IPMN progression to malignancy has been reported to be 2–3 % (Lévy et al. 2006; Kang et al. 2011). The details are described in a previous chapter.

14.2.2.2 Miscellaneous

Factors predictive of malignancy, along with the natural history of these lesions, are most important in determining whether surgery is indicated. However, other factors should be considered, including patient age, reflecting life expectancy; general condition making a patient suitable for major surgery; patient desire for a cure; and tumor location.

It has been proposed that for patients younger than 65 years old, a threshold of 2 cm be used to determine surgical resection because of the cumulative effect of cancer risk during the patients' lifetime (Weinberg et al. 2010; Farrell and Fernández-Del Castillo 2013). Although patients in different countries have shown marked discrepancies in life expectancy, in general, aggressive treatments should be recommended for patients likely to live more than 20 years, even if their cystic lesions are small (<3 cm).

Improvements in minimally invasive techniques have made laparoscopic distal pancreatectomy the standard treatment for most patients with benign and borderline pancreatic diseases, rather than pancreatoduodenectomy. More invasive surgical methods should be considered for tumors located in the body and/or tail of the pancreas.

14.3 Clinical Recommendations for Timing of Surgery

Due to the complexity of decision making required for patients with BD-IPMN, standard treatment guidelines applicable to every patient with BD-IPMN are not feasible. Rather, it is necessary to customize detailed treatment principles according to the clinical situation of each individual patient with BD-IPMN.

From a general perspective, the second consensus guidelines of the International Association of Pancreatology may be applicable to patients with IPMN (Tanaka et al. 2012) (Fig. 14.3). Although these guidelines had a low positive predictive value, despite a high negative predictive value, they provided specific and updated recommendations for resection and surveillance for BD-IPMN based on current evidence (Farrell and Fernández-Del Castillo 2013). Additional studies of patients with BD-IPMN may result in changes in clinical guidelines that more specifically consider individual risk factors.

References

Akita H, Takeda Y, Hoshino H, et al. Mural nodule in branch duct-type intraductal papillary mucinous neoplasms of the pancreas is a marker of malignant transformation and indication for surgery. Am J Surg. 2011;202:214–9.

Anand N, Sampath K, Wu BU. Cyst features and risk of malignancy in intraductal papillary mucinous neoplasms of the pancreas: a meta-analysis. Clin Gastroenterol Hepatol. 2013;11:913–21.

Arlix A, Bournet B, Otal P, et al. Long-term clinical and imaging follow-up of nonoperated branch duct form of intraductal papillary mucinous neoplasms of the pancreas. Pancreas. 2012;41:295–301.

Chiu SS, Lim JH, Lee WJ, Chang KT, Oh DK, Lee KT, et al. Intraductal papillary mucinous tumour of the pancreas: differentiation of malignancy and benignancy by CT. Clin Radiol. 2006;61:776–83.

Farrell JJ, Fernández-Del Castillo C. Pancreatic cystic neoplasms: management and unanswered questions. Gastroenterology. 2013;144:1303–15.

Ferrone CR, Finkelstein DM, Thayer SP, Muzikansky A, Fernandez-del Castillo C, Warshaw AL. Perioperative CA19-9 levels can predict stage and survival in patients with resectable pancreatic adenocarcinoma. J Clin Oncol. 2006;24:2897–902.

Fritz S, Hackert T, Hinz U, Hartwig W, Büchler MW, Werner J. Role of serum carbohydrate antigen 19-9 and carcinoembryonic antigen in distinguishing between benign and invasive intraductal papillary mucinous neoplasm of the pancreas. Br J Surg. 2011;98:104–10.

Fritz S, Klauss M, Bergmann F, Hackert T, Hartwig W, Strobel O, et al. Small (Sendai negative) branch-duct IPMNs: not harmless. Ann Surg. 2012;256:313–20.

Genevay M, Mino-Kenudson M, Yaeger K, Konstantinidis IT, Ferrone CR, Thayer S, et al. Cytology adds value to imaging studies for risk assessment of malignancy in pancreatic mucinous cysts. Ann Surg. 2011;254:977–83.

Hirono S, Tani M, Kawai M, Okada K, Miyazawa M, Shimizu A, et al. The carcinoembryonic antigen level in pancreatic juice and mural nodule size are predictors of malignancy for branch duct type intraductal papillary mucinous neoplasms of the pancreas. Ann Surg. 2012;255:517–22.

Hwang DW, Jang JY, Lim CS, Lee SE, Yoon YS, Ahn YJ, et al. Determination of malignant and invasive predictors in branch duct type intraductal papillary mucinous neoplasms of the pancreas: a suggested scoring formula. J Korean Med Sci. 2011;26:740–6.

Imaoka H, Yamao K, Salem AA, Mizuno N, Takahashi K, Sawaki A, et al. Pseudomyxoma peritonei caused by acute pancreatitis in intraductal papillary mucinous carcinoma of the pancreas. Pancreas. 2006;32:223–4.

Jang JY, Kim SW, Lee SE, Yang SH, Lee KU, Lee YJ, et al. Treatment guidelines for branch duct type intraductal papillary mucinous neoplasms of the pancreas: when can we operate or observe? Ann Surg Oncol. 2008;15:199–205.

Kang MJ, Jang JY, Kim SJ, Lee KB, Ryu JK, Kim YT, et al. Cyst growth rate predicts malignancy in patients with branch duct intraductal papillary mucinous neoplasms. Clin Gastroenterol Hepatol. 2011;9:87–93.

Lévy P, Jouannaud V, O'Toole D, Couvelard A, Vullierme MP, Palazzo L, et al. Natural history of intraductal papillary mucinous tumors of the pancreas: actuarial risk of malignancy. Clin Gastroenterol Hepatol. 2006;4:460–8.

Longnecker DS, Adsay NV, Fernandez-del Castillo C, Hruban RH, Kasugai T, Klimstra DS, et al. Histopathological diagnosis of pancreatic intraepithelial neoplasia and intraductal papillary-mucinous neoplasms: interobserver agreement. Pancreas. 2005;31:344–9.

Nagai K, Doi R, Ito T, et al. Single-institution validation of the international consensus guidelines for treatment of branch duct intraductal papillary mucinous neoplasms of the pancreas. J Hepatobiliary Pancreat Surg. 2009;16:353–8.

Ohno E, Itoh A, Kawashima H, Ishikawa T, Matsubara H, Itoh Y, et al. Malignant transformation of branch duct-type intraductal papillary mucinous neoplasms of the pancreas based on contrast-enhanced endoscopic ultrasonography morphological changes: focus on malignant transformation of intraductal papillary mucinous neoplasm itself. Pancreas. 2012;41:855–62.

Rautou PE, Lévy P, Vullierme MP, O'Toole D, Couvelard A, Cazals-Hatem D, et al. Morphologic changes in branch duct intraductal papillary mucinous neoplasms of the pancreas: a midterm follow-up study. Clin Gastroenterol Hepatol. 2008;6:807–14.

Rodriguez JR, Salvia R, Crippa S, et al. Branch-duct intraductal papillary mucinous neoplasms: observations in 145 patients who underwent resection. Gastroenterology. 2007;133:72–9.

Salvia R, Crippa S, Falconi M, Bassi C, Guarise A, Scarpa A, et al. Branch-duct intraductal papillary mucinous neoplasms of the pancreas: to operate or not to operate? Gut. 2007;56:1086–90.

Shimizu Y, Yamaue H, Maguchi H, Yamao K, Hirono S, Osanai M, et al. Predictors of malignancy in intraductal papillary mucinous neoplasm of the pancreas: analysis of 310 pancreatic resection patients at multiple high-volume centers. Pancreas. 2013;42:883–8.

Tanaka M, Chari S, Adsay V, Fernandez-del Castillo C, Falconi M, Shimizu M, et al. International consensus guidelines for management of intraductal papillary mucinous neoplasms and mucinous cystic neoplasms of the pancreas. Pancreatology. 2006;6:17–32.

Tanaka M, Fernández-del Castillo C, Adsay V, Chari S, Falconi M, Jang JY, et al. International consensus guidelines 2012 for the management of IPMN and MCN of the pancreas. Pancreatology. 2012;12:183–97.

Uehara H, Ishikawa O, Katayama K, Kawada N, Ikezawa K, Fukutake N, et al. Size of mural nodule as an indicator of surgery for branch duct intraductal papillary mucinous neoplasm of the pancreas during follow-up. J Gastroenterol. 2011;46:657–63.

Weinberg BM, Spiegel BM, Tomlinson JS, Farrell JJ. Asymptomatic pancreatic cystic neoplasms: maximizing survival and quality of life using Markov-based clinical nomograms. Gastroenterology. 2010;138:531–40.

Yamashita Y, Ueda K, Itonaga M, Yoshida T, Maeda H, Maekita T, et al. Usefulness of contrast-enhanced endoscopic sonography for discriminating mural nodules from mucous clots in intraductal papillary mucinous neoplasms: a single-center prospective study. J Ultrasound Med. 2013;32:61–8.

Zhong N, Zhang L, Takahashi N, et al. Histologic and imaging features of mural nodules in mucinous pancreatic cysts. Clin Gastroenterol Hepatol. 2012;10:192–8.

Chapter 15
Postoperative Surveillance of Main Duct IPMN

Takao Ohtsuka and Masao Tanaka

Abstract Surveillance schedule after resection of main duct IPMNs (MD-IPMNs) is determined based on pathological grade and surgical margin status. Prognosis after resection of invasive IPMNs is better than that of conventional pancreatic ductal adenocarcinomas (PDACs) in the matched status of T1 or N0, or the subtype of colloid carcinoma, while it is not different from that of PDACs in the other conditions (T2 to T4, N1, or other subtypes of carcinoma). Thus, the patients with invasive MD-IPMNs should be basically surveyed according to the protocol of the PDACs. In noninvasive IPMNs (low- to intermediate-grade dysplasia), if there is no residual lesion in the remnant pancreas with negative surgical margin, then the patients might be surveyed at 2 and 5 years after operation to check the development of new lesions in the remnant pancreas. In the patients having positive surgical margin of low- to intermediate-grade dysplasia, the surveillance of twice a year using physical examination and magnetic resonance imaging (MRI) might be suitable, although there has been no evidence regarding the effect of this protocol. On the other hand, it remains unclear whether this surveillance protocol of twice a year would be also applied to the patients after resection for noninvasive carcinoma (high-grade dysplasia). If there are some clinical signs to suspect the progression of the diseases in such patients, then surveillance with shorter interval is recommended.

Keywords IPMN • Main duct IPMN • Postoperative surveillance

T. Ohtsuka (✉) • M. Tanaka
Department of Surgery and Oncology, Graduate School of Medical Sciences, Kyushu University, Fukuoka, Japan
e-mail: takao-o@med.kyushu-u.ac.jp

M. Tanaka (ed.), *Intraductal Papillary Mucinous Neoplasm of the Pancreas*,
DOI 10.1007/978-4-431-54472-2_15, © Springer Japan 2014

15.1 Characteristics of Main Duct IPMN Relevant to Postoperative Surveillance

The mean rates of malignancy and invasive carcinoma in main duct IPMNs (MD-IPMNs) are 61.6 % and 43.1 %, respectively, and they are higher than those in branch duct IPMNs (BD-IPMNs) (25.5 % and 17.7 %, respectively) (Tanaka et al. 2012). As a result, postoperative prognosis of MD-IPMNs including any pathological grade is worse than that of BD-IPMNs (Serikawa et al. 2006; Nagai et al. 2008; Hwang et al. 2012). On the other hand, Massachusetts General Hospital and University of Verona group (Salvia et al. 2004) have shown that 10-year disease-specific survival rate of noninvasive MD-IPMNs after resection is 100 %, and there is no difference in postoperative survival rate between MD-IPMNs and BD-IPMNs when focusing on invasive carcinoma. Therefore, MD-IPMNs and BD-IPMNs may have the same malignant behavior in the matched pathological grade (Sohn et al. 2004; White et al. 2007; Partelli et al. 2010). One of the important factors to affect prognosis of invasive IPMNs after resection is pathological subtype, namely, gastric, intestinal, pancreatobiliary, and oncocytic. Several reports have shown that invasive carcinoma derived from intestinal subtype (colloid carcinoma) has better postoperative survival rate than that from non-intestinal subtype (tubular carcinoma or others) (Sohn et al. 2004; Poultsides et al. 2010; Sadakari et al. 2010; Furukawa et al. 2011; Mino-Kenudson et al. 2011; Yopp et al. 2011). Of notes, Furukawa et al. (2011) have recently reported that intestinal subtype is more frequently observed in MD-IPMNs than in other subtypes.

BD-IPMN often has multicentric lesions with 25–41 % of the prevalence (Tanaka et al. 2012), while most of the MD-IPMNs are of single lesion (Matthaei et al. 2012). Instead, MD-IPMNs have a tendency to spread along the main pancreatic duct and sometimes require additional resection during partial pancreatectomy or finally total pancreatectomy (Okada et al. 2010). Surgical margin status after partial pancreatectomy for IPMNs is an important factor for local recurrence (White et al. 2007), and therefore, international consensus guidelines (Tanaka et al. 2012) recommend obtaining a negative result or low- to intermediate-grade dysplasia at the pancreatic cut margin by intraoperative frozen section during partial pancreatectomy for IPMNs, while additional resection should be considered when high-grade dysplasia or invasive carcinoma is observed at the cut margin. Taken together, pathological grade and surgical margin status after partial pancreatectomy are important factors to influence to postoperative outcomes in patients with MD-IPMNs, and surveillance protocol should be considered based on these factors (Table 15.1).

15.2 Pathological Grade and Outcomes

Many reports (Chari et al. 2002; Wada et al. 2005; Partelli et al. 2010; Poultsides et al. 2010; Sadakari et al. 2010) have demonstrated the better postoperative prognosis of invasive IPMNs including both main duct and branch duct types than that

Table 15.1 Summary of characteristics of main duct IPMNs (MD-IPMNs) relevant to postoperative surveillance

1. Histological grade and outcomes
   a. The mean rates of malignancy and invasive carcinoma in MD-IPMNs are 61.6 % and 43.1 %, respectively
   b. Ten-year disease specific survival rate of noninvasive MD-IPMNs after resection is 100 %
   c. The postoperative survival rate of invasive IPMNs (30–60 %) is higher than 10–20 % of conventional pancreatic ductal adenocarcinomas
      - This is only limited in T1 or N0 status, and there is no difference in prognosis in T2 to T4 or N1 status
      - Invasive MD-IPMNs are frequently of intestinal subtype, of which subtype has better prognosis than other subtypes
2. Pancreatic margin status and local recurrence
   a. Most MD-IPMNs are of single lesion and have tendency to spread along the main pancreatic duct
   b. Significant lesions by frozen section are observed in 40 % of cases during pancreatectomy for MD-IPMNs
   c. Positive surgical margin status increases the rate of local recurrence (~20 %)
      - However, majority of the patients with positive margin status did not have local recurrence
      - Remnant total pancreatectomy for local recurrence of IPMNs leads to favorable prognosis

of conventional pancreatic ductal adenocarcinoma (PDAC); however, this is only limited in T1 or N0 status, and there is no difference in prognosis between invasive IPMNs and PDACs in T2 to T4 or N1 status (Poultsides et al. 2010). Morphological subtype is also the prognostic factor, and several reports have shown the better postoperative survival rate of invasive carcinoma derived from intestinal subtype (colloid carcinoma) than that of invasive carcinoma derived from non-intestinal subtype, as described above, and the prognosis of non-intestinal invasive IPMNs is almost same with that of PDACs (Sadakari et al. 2010; Furukawa et al. 2011). In invasive IPMNs, surgical margin status after partial pancreatectomy does not affect postoperative survival, because distant metastatic recurrence is more likely to affect patients' prognosis than local recurrence (Wada et al. 2005).

15.3 Surgical Margin Status and Outcomes

Pancreatic margin status during partial pancreatectomy for IPMNs is usually determined by the presence or absence of neoplastic cells of IPMNs; any grade of IPMNs including low-, intermediate-, and high-grade dysplasia as positive, and normal epithelia or low-grade pancreatic intraepitherial neoplasia (PanIN-1 or 2) as negative (Chari et al. 2002; White et al. 2007). On the other hand, positive results of pancreatic margin status by frozen sectioning during pancreatectomy would not be always an indication for additional resection, and it depends on the degree of the dysplasia. If there is high-grade dysplasia or invasive carcinoma at the pancreatic cut margin, then additional resection is recommended until obtaining a negative margin in international consensus guidelines (Tanaka et al. 2012), although it remains unclear whether the presence intermediate-grade dysplasia at surgical margin might influence postoperative postoperative outcomes and how to survey such patients in terms of surveillance interval and diagnostic modalities. Frozen sectioning of the pancreatic cut margin during partial pancreatectomy for IPMNs is reliable because its result is consistent with the final definitive examination in 94 % of the cases and it changes the extent of the resection in 30 % and leads adequate resection in 97 % of the patients (Couvelard et al. 2005). Of note, significant lesions at the first analysis of frozen section are more frequently observed during pancreatectomy for MD-IPMNs (40 %) than pancreatectomy for BD-IPMNs (14 %) (Couvelard et al. 2005), because of the characteristics of MD-IPMNs to spread laterally along the main pancreatic duct (Okada et al. 2010).

The rate of local recurrence in the remnant pancreas after resection of IPMNs is reported to be 0–20 % during initial postoperative 5 years (Chari et al. 2002; Wada et al. 2005; White et al. 2007), and positive surgical margin increases the rate of local recurrence (White et al. 2007). On the other hand, we sometimes experience recurrence in the remnant pancreas after partial pancreatectomy for IPMNs, even though the negative margin status at the initial operation (Fig. 15.1). There seems to be no difference in the rate of local recurrence after partial pancreatectomy between MD-IPMNs and BD-IPMNs (White et al. 2007), although it is unclear whether those might be metachronous development of new lesions, progression of residual lesions, or metastases of primary lesions. Although total pancreatectomy definitively prevents the local recurrence of IPMNs, most of the patients with positive margin status can survive without recurrence, and remnant total pancreatectomy for local recurrence of IPMNs leads to favorable prognosis (White et al. 2007). Therefore, prophylactic total pancreatectomy for IPMNs is not recommended at present.

There are several reports showing the details in recurrence in the remnant pancreas after resection of IPMNs. White et al. (2007) analyzed 78 patients with resected noninvasive IPMNs including both main duct and branch duct types and found that six patients (7.7 %) had recurrence in the remnant pancreas with a median interval of 22 months (range 8–62 months). The recurrence rate of positive margin status at initial operation (17 %, 4/23) was higher than that of negative margin status (2 %, 1/50); however, on the other hand, the majority of the patients (83 %) with positive margin status did not have local recurrence. Three of these six patients with recurrence could undergo curative remnant pancreatectomy. Chari et al. (2002) experienced five patients (6.8 %) having local recurrence in 73 resected noninvasive IPMNs with a median interval of 37 months (range 34–75), despite the surgical margin was negative at the initial operation. Salvia et al. (2004) showed that 8 (7 %) of 114 patients who underwent partial pancreatectomy for MD-IPMNs had local recurrence. One of them had pathologically noninvasive IMPN (adenoma) with negative margin at the initial operation, and the patient underwent completion pancreatectomy for recurrent noninvasive carcinoma 5 years after initial operation. The remaining seven patients had invasive IPMNs at initial operation, and three of them had positive margin, two had negative margin, and detail was unknown in the other two.

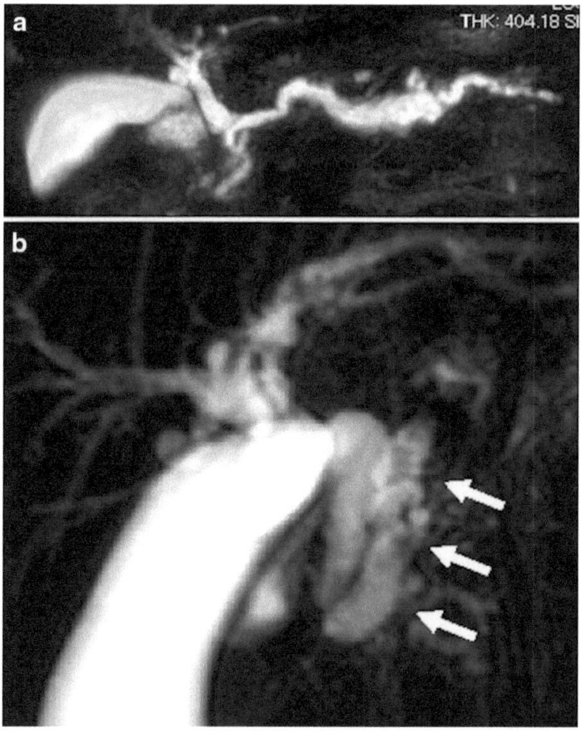

Fig. 15.1 Recurrence of IPMN in the remnant pancreas after resection of main duct IPMN. (**a**) Magnetic resonance cholangiopancreatography (MRCP) shows the dilation of the main pancreatic duct in the pancreatic body, and the diagnosis of main duct IPMN (MD-IPMN) was made. The patient underwent distal pancreatectomy, and the resected specimen demonstrated high-grade dysplasia of IPMN. Surgical cut margin showed low-grade dysplasia. (**b**) MRCP at 32 months after the initial operation demonstrates the dilation of the main pancreatic duct in the remnant pancreas (*arrows*). Pancreatic juice cytology under endoscopic retrograde pancreatography showed adenocarcinoma, and the patient subsequently underwent remnant total pancreatectomy. The resected specimen revealed IPMN with an associated invasive carcinoma

15.4 Surveillance Protocol After Resection of MD-IPMNs

Regarding postoperative surveillance based on pathological grade and pancreatic margin status, the protocol is almost the same between MD-IPMNs and BD-IPMNs, while in BD-IPMNs, additional factors such as multicentric occurrence of BD-IPMNs or progression of the residual lesions in the remnant pancreas and development of concomitant PDACs should be considered. One example of surveillance protocol after resection of MD-IPMNs is presented in Fig. 15.2.

The prognosis of invasive IPMNs after resection is significantly but slightly better than that of conventional PDACs, and therefore, surveillance protocol of invasive IPMNs after resection should follow the protocol of conventional PDACs.

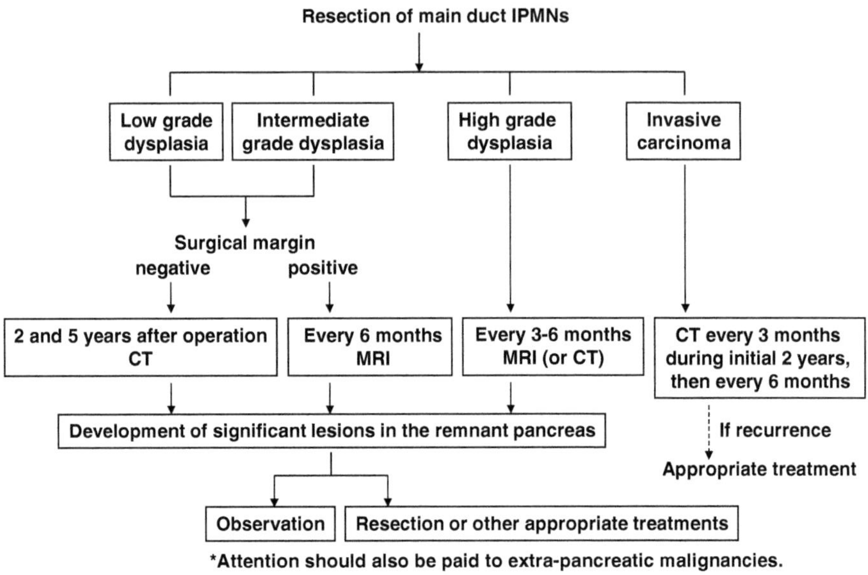

Fig. 15.2 One example of surveillance protocol after resection of main duct IPMN

National Comprehensive Cancer Network (NCCN) Guidelines (2012) recommend the surveillance of the patients after resection of PDACs every 3–6 months for initial 2 years, then annually, using physical examinations, assessment of serum carbohydrate antigen 19-9 (CA19-9) level, and computed tomography (CT).

If there is no residual lesion in the remnant pancreas with negative surgical margin after resection for low- to intermediate-grade dysplasia of MD-IPMNs, the patients might be checked at 2 and 5 years after operation to check the development of new lesions in the remnant pancreas. In the patients having positive surgical margin of low- to intermediate-grade dysplasia, the surveillance of twice a year using physical examination and magnetic resonance imaging (MRI) might be suitable (Fig. 15.2). On the other hand, it remains unclear whether this surveillance protocol of twice a year would be also applied to the patients after resection for noninvasive carcinoma (high-grade dysplasia), because local recurrence of MD-IPMN seems to be more frequently observed after resection of high-grade dysplasia than after resection of low- to intermediate-grade dysplasia, despite the negative surgical margin status (Ohtsuka et al. 2012). If there are some clinical signs to suspect the progression of the diseases such as deterioration of diabetes, elevation of serum CA19-9, abdominal pain, and increase in diameter of pancreatic duct, then the surveillance of shorter interval is recommended.

We sometimes experience the patients having pancreatic ductal dilation after pancreaticoenterostomy followed by pancreas head resection for IPMNs, and it is often difficult to determine whether it might be caused by anastomotic stenosis or recurrence of IPMN. In this case, endoscopic retrograde pancreatography (ERP) might be useful because it allows the direct observation of the anastomosis and the collection of the pancreatic juice; however, endoscopic approach to the pancreatic anastomosis using regular ERP method is difficult, especially in Billroth-II type of the reconstruction. Inagaki et al. (1999) recommended the use of Billroth-I type reconstruction rather than Billroth-II type reconstruction following pancreatoduodenectomy for IPMNs for the postoperative assessment of the remnant pancreas by ERP. Kikuyama et al. (2012) have recently reported the usefulness of double-balloon endoscopy to assess the pancreatic anastomosis after Billroth-II type pancreatoduodenectomy.

Development of extrapancreatic malignancy is also reported in patients after resection of MD-IPMNs (Sugiyama and Atomi. 1999; Reid-Lombardo et al. 2010), and details of this issues including surveillance protocol have been described in another chapter (Chap. 10).

References

Chari ST, Yadav D, Smyrk TC, et al. Study of recurrence after surgical resection of intraductal papillary mucinous neoplasm of the pancreas. Gastroenterology. 2002;123:1500–7.

Couvelard A, Sauvanet A, Kainmanesh R, et al. Frozen sectioning of the pancreatic cut surface during resection of intraductal papillary mucinous neoplasms of the pancreas is useful and reliable. Ann Surg. 2005;242:774–80.

Furukawa T, Hatori T, Fujita I, et al. Prognostic relevance of morphological types of intraductal papillary mucinous neoplasms of the pancreas. Gut. 2011;60:509–16.

Hwang DW, Jang JY, Lee SE, et al. Clinicopathologic analysis of surgically proven intraductal papillary mucinous neoplasms of the pancreas in SNUH: a 15-year experience at a single academic institution. Langenbecks Arch Surg. 2012;397:93–102.

Inagaki M, Maguchi M, Kino S, et al. Mucin-producing tumors of the pancreas: clinicopathological features, surgical treatment, and outcome. J Hepatobiliary Pancreat Surg. 1999;6:281–5.

Kikuyama M, Itoi T, Ota Y, et al. Therapeutic endoscopy for stenotic pancreatodigestive tract anastomosis after pancreatoduodenectomy. Gastrointest Endosc. 2012;73:376–82.

Matthaei H, Norris AL, Tsiatis AC, et al. Clinicopathological characteristics and molecular analyses of multifocal intraductal papillary mucinous neoplasms of the pancreas. Ann Surg. 2012;255:326–33.

Mino-Kenudson M, Fernández-del Castillo C, Baba Y, et al. Prognosis of invasive intraductal papillary mucinous neoplasm depends on histological and precursor epithelial subtypes. Gut. 2011;60:1712–20.

Nagai K, Doi R, Kida A, et al. Intraductal papillary mucinous neoplasms of the pancreas: clinicopathologic characteristics and long-term follow-up after resection. World J Surg. 2008;32:271–8.

NCCN clinical practice guidelines in oncology (NCCN Guidelines ™). Pancreatic adenocarcinoma. Version I 2012. 2012. http://www.nccn.org.

Ohtsuka T, Kono H, Tanabe R, et al. Follow-up study after resection of intraductal papillary mucinous neoplasm of the pancreas: special references to the multifocal lesions and development of ductal carcinoma in the remnant pancreas. Am J Surg. 2012;204:44–8.

Okada K, Imaizumi T, Hirabayashi K, et al. The distance of the tumor spread in the main pancreatic duct of an intraductal papillary-mucinous neoplasm: where to resect and how to predict it. J Hepatobiliary Pancreat Sci. 2010;17:516–22.

Partelli S, Fernández-del Castillo C, Bassi C, et al. Invasive intraductal papillary mucinous carcinomas of the pancreas. Predictors of survival and the role of lymph node ratio. Ann Surg. 2010;251:477–82.

Poultsides GA, Reddy S, Cameron JL, et al. Histopathologic basis for the favorable survival after resection of intraductal papillary mucinous neoplasm-associated invasive adenocarcinoma of the pancreas. Ann Surg. 2010;251:470–6.
Reid-Lombardo KM, Mathis KL, Wood CM, et al. Frequency of extrapancreatic neoplasms in intraductal papillary mucinous neoplasm of the pancreas. Implication for management. Ann Surg. 2010;251:64–9.
Sadakari Y, Ohuchida K, Nakata K, et al. Invasive carcinoma derived from non-intestinal type intraductal papillary mucinous neoplasm of the pancreas has a poorer prognosis than that derived from intestinal type. Surgery. 2010;147:812–7.
Salvia R, Fernández-del Castillo C, Bassi C, et al. Main-duct intraductal papillary mucinous neoplasms of the pancreas. Clinical predictors of malignancy and long-term survival following resection. Ann Surg. 2004;239:678–87.
Serikawa M, Sasaki T, Fujimoto Y, et al. Management of intraductal papillary-mucinous neoplasm of the pancreas: treatment strategy based on morphologic classification. J Clin Gastroenterol. 2006;40:856–62.
Sohn TA, Yeo CJ, Cameron JL, et al. Intraductal papillary mucinous neoplasms of the pancreas. An updated experience. Ann Surg. 2004;239:788–99.
Sugiyama M, Atomi Y. Extrapancreatic neoplasms occur with unusual frequency in patients with intraductal papillary mucinous tumors of the pancreas. Am J Gastroenterol. 1999;94:470–3.
Tanaka M, Fernández-del Castillo C, Adsay V, et al. International consensus guidelines 2012 for the management of IPMN and MCN of the pancreas. Pancreatology. 2012;12:183–97.
Wada K, Kozarek RA, Traverso LW. Outcomes following resection of invasive and noninvasive intraductal papillary mucinous neoplasms of the pancreas. Am J Surg. 2005;189:632–7.
White R, D'Angelica M, Katabi N, et al. Fate of the remnant pancreas after resection of noninvasive intraductal papillary mucinous neoplasm. J Am Coll Surg. 2007;204:987–95.
Yopp AC, Katabi N, Janakos M, et al. Invasive carcinoma arising in intraductal papillary mucinous neoplasms of the pancreas. A match control study with conventional pancreatic ductal adenocarcinoma. Ann Surg. 2011;253:968–74.

Chapter 16
Postoperative Surveillance of Branch Duct IPMN

Takao Ohtsuka and Masao Tanaka

Abstract Surveillance protocol after resection of branch duct IPMNs (BD-IPMNs) is determined based on the following factors: (1) pathological grade of resected BD-IPMNs, (2) pancreatic margin status after partial pancreatectomy, (3) presence of the residual lesions left without resection in the remnant pancreas, (4) presence of concomitant PDACs at the time of operation, (5) the possibility of metachronous occurrence of BD-IPMNs, and (6) development of concomitant PDACs in the remnant pancreas. Yearly risk of PDAC development is reported to be 0.7–0.9 % in the patients with BD-IPMNs, and thus international consensus guidelines suggest that CT or MRCP at 6-month intervals is appropriate for surveillance after resection of BD-IPMNs, even though the resected IPMN is benign with negative surgical margin. Surveillance with shorter interval should be considered in patients who underwent resection of invasive IPMNs, who had positive surgical margin status, or who have significant clinical signs to suspect the progression or new development of the disease.

Keywords Branch duct IPMN • IPMN • Postoperative surveillance

16.1 Characteristics of Branch Duct IPMNs Relevant to Postoperative Surveillance

Most of the branch duct IPMNs (BD-IPMNs) are benign, which do not have any malignancy predictors described in the international consensus guidelines (Tanaka et al. 2012). Even in the resected lesions which have several malignancy predictors, malignant BD-IPMNs are observed in only 25.5 %, which is lower than 61.6 % of

T. Ohtsuka (✉) • M. Tanaka
Department of Surgery and Oncology, Graduate School of Medical Sciences, Kyushu University, Fukuoka, Japan
e-mail: takao-o@med.kyushu-u.ac.jp

M. Tanaka (ed.), *Intraductal Papillary Mucinous Neoplasm of the Pancreas*,
DOI 10.1007/978-4-431-54472-2_16,

main duct IPMNs (MD-IPMNs) (Tanaka et al. 2012). Thus, malignant potential of BD-IPMNs is lower than that of MD-IPMNs; however, there seems to be no difference in postoperative prognosis between noninvasive MD-IPMNs and noninvasive BD-IPMNs, or between invasive MD-IPMNs and invasive BD-IPMNs (Sohn et al. 2004; White et al. 2007; Partelli et al. 2010).

Most MD-IPMNs are of single lesion having tendency to spread laterally along main pancreatic duct, while 25–41 % of BD-IPMNs have multiple lesions which develop independently of each other (Matthaei et al. 2012; Okada et al. 2010; Tanaka et al. 2012). Thus, negative pancreatic cut margin can be more easily obtained after partial pancreatectomy for BD-IPMNs than that after MD-IPMNs (Couvelard et al. 2005). In multiple BD-IPMNs, international consensus guidelines suggest to resect only the lesion having some malignancy predictor while to leave the lesions without any malignancy predictor in the remnant pancreas for avoiding total pancreatectomy; however, careful attention should be paid to the possible progression of residual lesions left in the remnant pancreas and new development of the BD-IPMNs in the remnant pancreas (Tanaka et al. 2012).

Another important issue is the synchronous or metachronous occurrence of pancreatic ductal adenocarcinomas (PDACs) concomitant with BD-IPMNs, and prevalence of concomitant PDACs is reported to be 2.0–9.9 % of the patients with BD-IPMNs including both resected and observed lesions (Yamaguchi et al. 2002; Tada et al. 2006; Uehara et al. 2008; Sawai et al. 2010; Ingkakul et al. 2010; Tanno et al. 2010a; Tanno et al. 2010b; Maguchi et al. 2011; Yamaguchi et al. 2011; Ohtsuka et al. 2012).

Taken together, surveillance protocol after resection of BD-IPMNs should be considered based on the following factors: (1) pathological grade of resected BD-IPMNs, (2) pancreatic margin status after partial pancreatectomy, (3) presence of the residual lesions left without resection in the remnant pancreas, (4) presence of concomitant PDACs at the time of operation, (5) the possibility of metachronous occurrence of BD-IPMNs, and (6) development of concomitant PDACs in the remnant pancreas during surveillance.

16.2 Pathological Grade and Outcomes

Disease-specific survival rate of noninvasive and invasive BD-IPMNs are 100 % and 63 %, respectively (Rodriguez et al. 2007), which are same with 100 % and 60 % of MD-IPMNs, respectively (Salvia et al. 2004). The reported postoperative survival rates of invasive IPMNs (30–60 %) seem to be higher than 10–20 % of conventional PDACs (Chari et al. 2002; Wada et al. 2005; Partelli et al. 2010; Poultsides et al. 2010; Sadakari et al. 2010; Yopp et al. 2011). One of the reasons is that many of invasive IPMNs are of colloid carcinomas derived from intestinal subtype, which have better prognosis than invasive carcinomas derived from other subtypes (Sadakari et al. 2010; Mino-Kenudson et al. 2011; Furukawa et al. 2011). The other reason is the pathological stage at the time of resection, and Yamaguchi et al. (2011) have analyzed 765 patients who underwent resection of BD-IPMNs in a Japanese multicenter study and found that invasive IPMNs were diagnosed earlier than conventional PDACs. On the other hand, Poultsides et al. (2010) have recently showed that postoperative prognosis of invasive IPMNs is better than that of PDACs in matched T1 or N0 status, while there was no difference in the prognosis between these two entities in T2 to T4 or N1 status and, therefore, concluded that advanced invasive IPMNs have the same malignant behavior as conventional PDACs.

16.3 Surgical Margin Status and Outcomes

Although intraepithelial spread along the main pancreatic duct is observed in about half of the patients who underwent resection of BD-IPMNs, the reported length of the tumor spread is not so long (mean, 25.2 mm) (Kobayashi et al. 2011). As a result, a negative surgical margin is more easily obtained during partial pancreatectomy for BD-IPMNs, compared with MD-IPMNs (Couvelard et al. 2005). A positive surgical margin increases the rate of local recurrence; however, the majority of the patients with a positive margin can survive without recurrence, and remnant total pancreatectomy leads to favorable prognosis even in patients having local recurrence (White et al. 2007). Thus, in terms of the surgical margin status, the goal during pancreatectomy is to obtain negative or low- to intermediate-grade dysplasia at pancreatic cut margin by frozen sectioning, as described in the international consensus guidelines (Tanaka et al. 2012). More details regarding this issue are described in the other chapter (Chap. 14, Sect. 3).

16.4 Outcomes of the Residual Lesions Left Without Resection in the Remnant Pancreas

Few data are available on the outcomes of residual lesions after resection of multifocal BD-IPMNs; however, Mori et al. (2012) have recently analyzed the surveillance data of 211 patients with BD-IPMNs, including 69 who underwent resection, and demonstrated that 13 BD-IPMNs left in the remnant pancreas after partial pancreatectomy in 11 patients did not show any morphological change during mean follow-up period of 30 months. The mean size of 13 lesions was 15 mm, and those lesions did not have any malignancy predictors. They also found that there is no difference in the prevalence of concomitant PDACs or prognosis between solitary and multifocal BD-IPMNs. Basically, clinical characteristics of multifocal BD-IPMNs are not different from those of solitary BD-IPMNs, and surgery does not seem to alter the oncological characteristics of BD-IPMN left in the remnant pancreas. The international consensus guidelines (Tanaka et al. 2012) suggest to manage the BD-IPMNs left in the remnant pancreas without any malignancy predictors as those observed without resection (See Chap. 3).

16.5 Metachronous Development of BD-IPMNs

Rodriguez et al. (2007) experienced four patients (3 %) having metachronous occurrence of IPMNs in the remnant pancreas after mean follow-up period of 34.7 months in 145 patients who underwent resection of BD-IPMNs. All four patients had benign IPMN (adenoma) at the initial operation with a negative surgical cut margin. Ohtsuka et al. (2012) reported that six metachronous development of BD-IPMNs (5 %) were observed in 128 patients who underwent resection of BD-IPMNs, after a mean of 23 postoperative months. All the patients in these two reports were asymptomatic at the time of the diagnosis of metachronous BD-IPMNs, and all those lesions were of less than 30 mm in size without any other malignancy predictors and did not require resection. Therefore, metachronous development of BD-IPMNs in the remnant pancreas is not frequently observed, and even though such lesions occur, they are indolent.

16.6 Metachronous Development of Concomitant PDACs

Most of the IPMNs having concomitant PDACs are of branch duct type, and majority of the distinct PDACs are diagnosed synchronously at the initial assessment of IPMNs or during surveillance of BD-IPMNs observed without resection (Yamaguchi et al. 2002; Tada et al. 2006; Uehara et al. 2008; Sawai et al. 2010; Ingkakul et al. 2010; Tanno et al. 2010a; Tanno et al. 2010b; Maguchi et al. 2011; Yamaguchi et al. 2011; Ohtsuka et al. 2012). On the other hand, few data are available on the metachronous development of distinct PDACs during postoperative surveillance of IPMNs. Our group (Ohtsuka et al. 2013) has recently reported that a total of 23 PDACs developed in 20 of 179 patients (11.2 %) who underwent resection of IPMNs, and 16 of 23 lesions were synchronous and the 7 were metachronous (three patients had both synchronous and metachronous lesions) (Fig. 16.1). Twenty of the twenty-three lesions were resected, while the remaining three were unresectable because of hepatic metastases. The interval between the initial operation for IPMNs and the diagnosis of metachronous PDACs in seven patients ranged from 1 to 15 years, indicating necessity of long-term surveillance for more than 10 years. Of note, seven metachronous PDACs including three unresectable diseases were diagnosed at a more advanced stage than synchronous PDACs. One of the reasons considered for the delay in the diagnosis of metachronous PDACs is that sensitive diagnostic modalities for early detection of concomitant PDACs such as endoscopic retrograde pancreatography (ERP) and endoscopic ultrasonography (EUS) are difficult to be applied for the patients after pancreatectomy (especially pancreatoduodenectomy) because of the anatomical deformity. In addition, surveillance protocol for early detection of PDACs during management of BD-IPMNs has not been determined in terms of interval, duration, and diagnostic modalities.

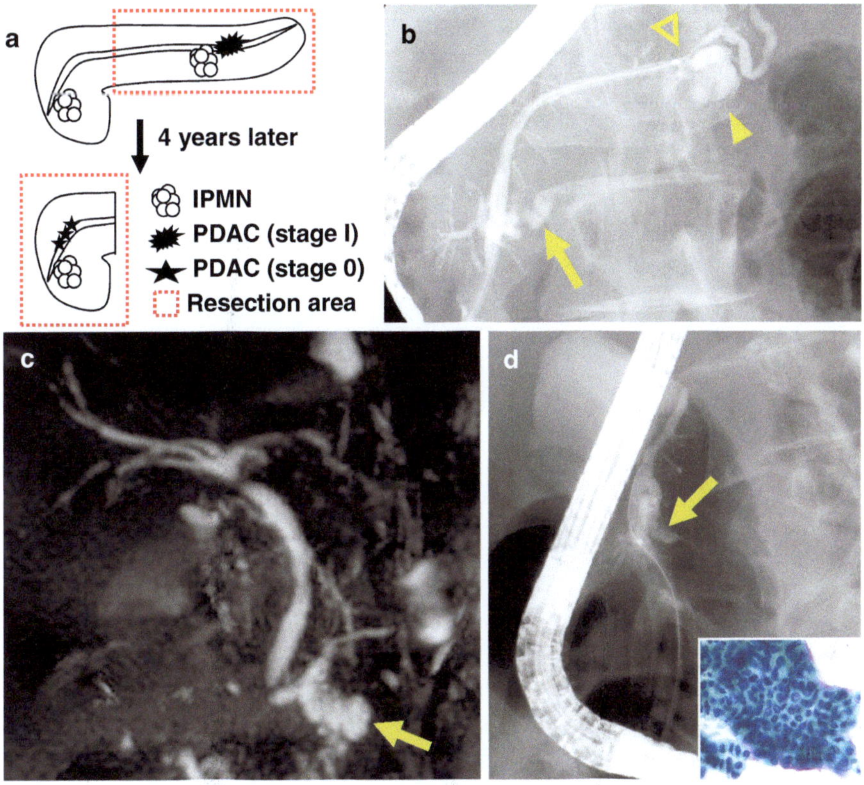

Fig. 16.1 Resectable case of synchronous and metachronous concomitant pancreatic ductal adenocarcinomas. (**a**) Schema of the clinical course of the patient. The patient underwent distal pancreatectomy for low-grade dysplasia of BD-IPMN and distinct pancreatic ductal adenocarcinoma (PDAC) [stage I according to the Japanese classification of pancreatic carcinoma (Japan Pancreas Society. 2011)] in the distal pancreas. BD-IPMN in the pancreas head without any malignancy predictors was left without operation. Four years after the initial operation, the patient underwent remnant total pancreatectomy because of positive result of pancreatic juice cytology. The pathology of resected specimen indicated noninvasive PDAC (stage 0) in the main pancreatic duct and intermediate-grade dysplasia of residual BD-IPMN. (**b**) Endoscopic retrograde pancreatography (ERP) at the time of initial operation demonstrates the cystic lesions in the head (*arrow*) and body (*closed arrowhead*) of the pancreas which communicate with main pancreatic duct and irregular stenosis of main pancreatic duct in the pancreas body (*open arrowhead*). (**c**) Magnetic resonance cholangiopancreatography (MRCP) at the time of metachronous development of noninvasive PDAC demonstrates no morphological change of residual BD-IPMN (*arrow*) as well as no abnormality in the main pancreatic duct. (**d**) ERP also shows cystic lesion (*arrow*) in the remnant pancreas, but no abnormality in the main pancreatic duct. However, pancreatic juice cytology revealed adenocarcinoma (*right lower panel*), and thus the remnant total pancreatectomy was performed

16.7 Surveillance Protocol After Resection of BD-IPMNs

We sometimes experience the patients having metachronous occurrence of BD-IPMNs in the remnant pancreas; however, those lesions were usually indolent. Residual BD-IPMNs left in the remnant pancreas after resection of primary lesion also show no morphological change during long-term postoperative surveillance period (Fig. 16.2). The effect of these two factors on postoperative outcomes after

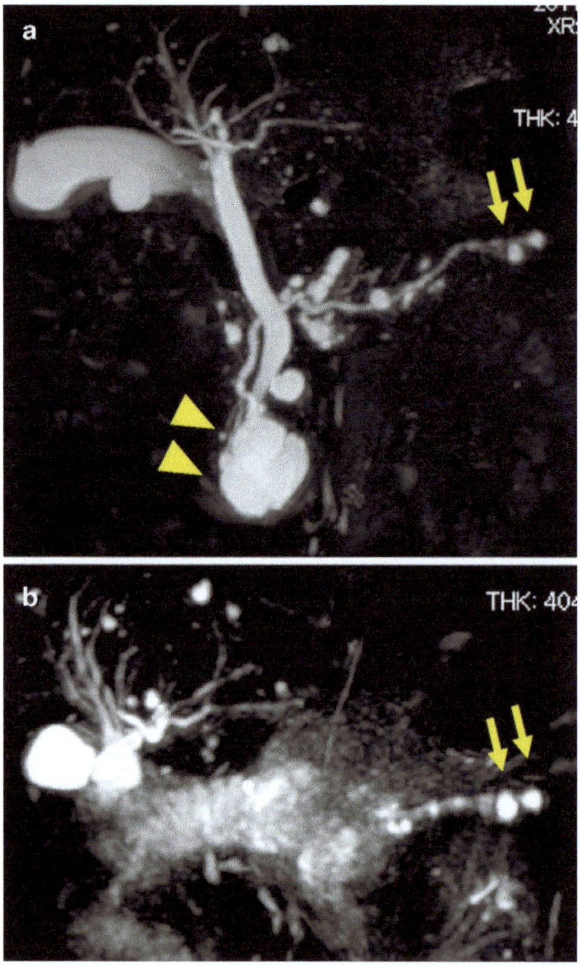

Fig. 16.2 Follow-up imaging after resection of multiple branch duct IPMNs. (**a**) Magnetic resonance cholangiopancreatography (MRCP) demonstrates multiple branch duct IPMNs (BD-IPMNs). The patient underwent pancreatoduodenectomy including the resection of BD-IPMN in the pancreas head (*arrowhead*) and small BD-IPMNs in the pancreas head and body, while the small cysts in the pancreas tail (*arrow*) were left without resection. (**b**) MRCP at 1 year after the operation shows that the residual lesions in the remnant pancreas do not present morphological change (*arrows*)

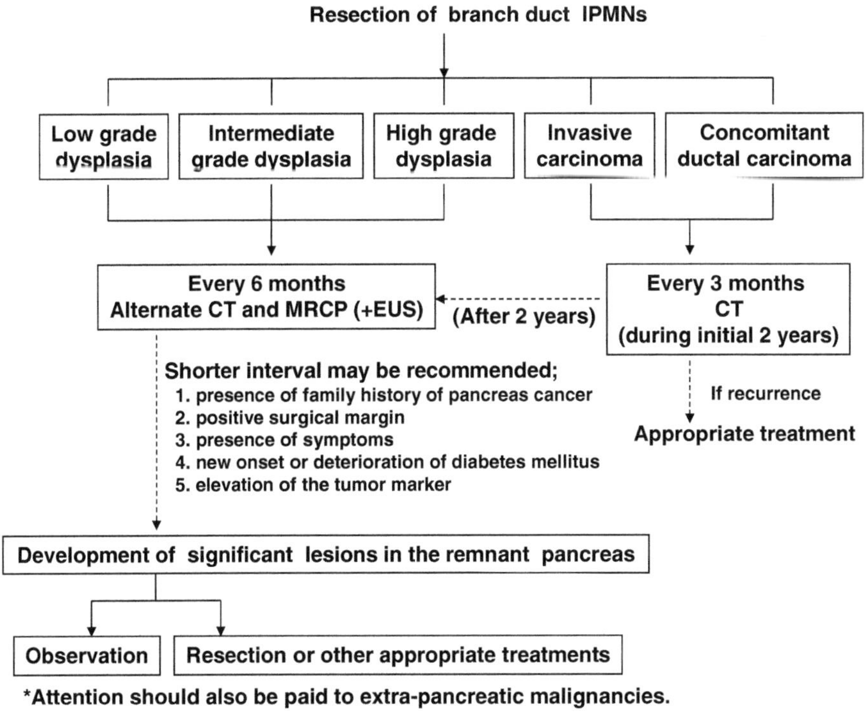

Fig. 16.3 One example of surveillance protocol after resection of branch duct IPMNs

resection of BD-IPMNs is limited. The most important issue after resection of BD-IPMNs is the development of concomitant PDACs. Yearly risk of PDAC development is reported to be 0.7–0.9 % in the patients with BD-IPMNs, and therefore international consensus guidelines suggest that CT or MRCP at 6-month intervals is appropriate for surveillance after resection of BD-IPMNs, even though the resected IPMN is noninvasive with negative surgical margin (Tanaka et al. 2012). Of course, shorter-interval surveillance should be considered in patients undergoing resection of invasive IPMNs, having positive surgical margin status, or presenting significant clinical signs such as symptoms, morphological change of the residual lesion, deterioration of diabetes, and elevation of tumor markers (Tanaka et al. 2012). One example of surveillance protocol after resection of MD-IPMNs is presented in Fig. 16.3.

On the other hand, we have recently experienced a patient who was diagnosed as having unresectable PDACs despite the surveillance of 6 months interval after resection of BD-IPMN (Fig. 16.4). Thus, EUS and ERP in addition to CT and MRCP might be required for early detection of metachronous development of concomitant PDACs, although indication and timing of these modalities remain controversial in patients after resection of BD-IPMNs.

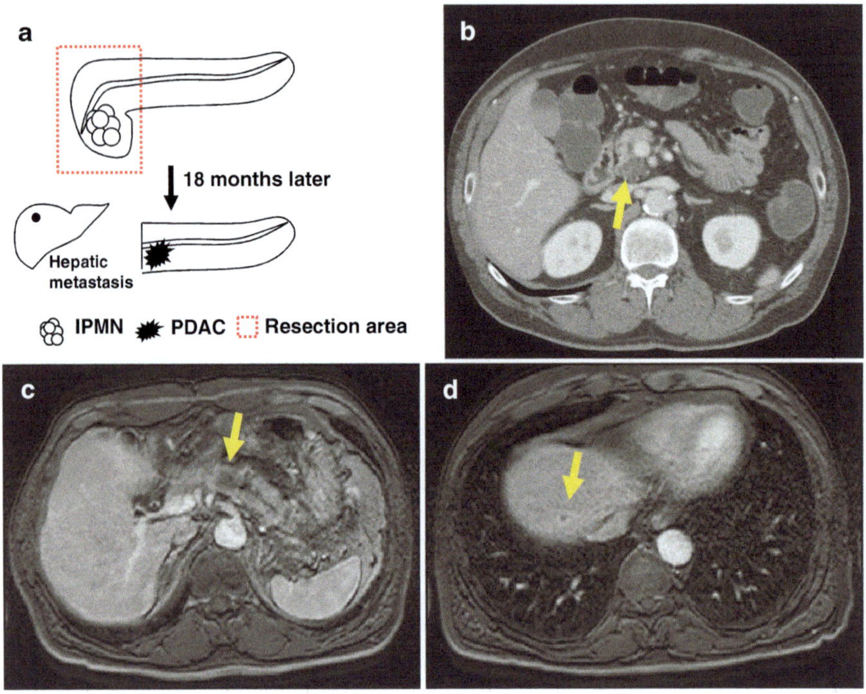

Fig. 16.4 Unresectable case of metachronous development of pancreatic ductal adenocarcinoma after resection of branch duct IPMN. (**a**) Schema of the clinical course of the patient. The patient underwent pancreatoduodenectomy for high-grade dysplasia of BD-IPMN in the pancreas head with negative surgical margin. Then the patient was surveyed by alternate CT and magnetic resonance imaging (MRI) at 6 months interval. However, the patient was diagnosed as having metachronous development of unresectable pancreatic ductal adenocarcinoma (PDAC) with hepatic metastasis. (**b**) Computed tomography (CT) at the time of operation for BD-IPMN demonstrates cystic lesions in the head of the pancreas (*arrow*), 25 mm in diameter, with slight dilation of main pancreatic duct. Preoperative pancreatic juice cytology revealed adenocarcinoma, and the patient underwent pancreatoduodenectomy. (**c**) MRI at 18 months after operation demonstrates delayed-enhanced solid mass (*arrow*), 20 mm in diameter, in the remnant pancreas near the pancreatojejunostomy and (**d**) ringed-enhanced lesion (*arrow*), 5 mm in diameter, in the right lobe of the liver. Endoscopic ultrasonography-guided fine needle aspiration cytology for pancreatic lesion revealed adenocarcinoma. The patient had episodes of the deterioration of diabetes mellitus and elevation of carbohydrate antigen 19-9 (CA19-9) at the time of diagnosis of metachronous PDAC. These findings have been reported to be predictive of the possible presence of concomitant PDAC in patients with branch duct IPMNs (Ingkakul et al. 2010)

We have also recently identified that the IPMNs having concomitant PDACs are characterized as showing gastric subtype of benign BD-IPMNs, in which *GNAS* gene mutation is rarely observed (Ideno et al. 2013). Therefore, strict surveillance of the patients who are found to have gastric subtype BD-IPMN without *GNAS* mutation during pathological assessment of resected specimen might lead to increased number of early detection of concomitant PDACs after resection of BD-IPMNs.

Table 16.1 Summary of characteristics of branch duct IPMNs (BD-IPMNs) relevant to postoperative surveillance

1. Histological grade and outcomes
   a. The mean rates of malignancy and invasive carcinoma in BD-IPMNs are 25.5 % and 17.7 %, respectively
   b. Ten-year disease specific survival rate of noninvasive BD-IPMNs after resection is 100 %
   c. There is no difference in postoperative survival rate between invasive main duct IPMNs and invasive BD-IPMNs
2. Pancreatic margin status and local recurrence
   a. Significant lesions by frozen section are rarely observed during pancreatectomy for BD-IPMNs
3. Presence of the residual lesions left without resection in the remnant pancreas
   a. The prevalence of multiple BD-IPMNs is 25–41 %
   b. In multiple BD-IPMNs, only the lesions having malignancy predictors are indication for resection. The lesions without malignancy predictor can be left in the remnant pancreas
   c. Most residual lesions do not show any morphological change during postoperative surveillance
4. Metachronous occurrence of BD-IPMNs in the remnant pancreas
   a. Not frequently observed. Even though such lesions occur, they are indolent
5. Pancreatic ductal adenocarcinoma (PDACs) concomitant with BD-IPMNs
   a. The prevalence, 2.0–11.2 %
   b. Majority of the concomitant PDACs are diagnosed synchronously during the initial assessment of or surveillance of BD-IPMNs
   c. The interval between the initial operation for IPMNs and the diagnosis of metachronous PDACs ranges from 1 to 15 years
   d. In some report, 80 % of concomitant PDACs are resectable
   e. Metachronous PDACs are diagnosed at a more advanced stage than synchronous PDACs

Development of extrapancreatic malignancy is also reported in patients after resection of BD-IPMNs as well as MD-IPMNs (Sugiyama and Atomi 1999; Reid-Lombardo et al. 2010), and details of these issues including surveillance protocol have been described in another chapter (Chap. 10) (Table 16.1).

References

Chari ST, Yadav D, Smyrk TC, et al. Study of recurrence after surgical resection of intraductal papillary mucinous neoplasm of the pancreas. Gastroenterology. 2002;123:1500–7.

Couvelard A, Sauvanet A, Kainmanesh R, et al. Frozen sectioning of the pancreatic cut surface during resection of intraductal papillary mucinous neoplasms of the pancreas is useful and reliable. Ann Surg. 2005;242:774–80.

Furukawa T, Hatori T, Fujita I, et al. Prognostic relevance of morphological types of intraductal papillary mucinous neoplasms of the pancreas. Gut. 2011;60:509–16.

Ideno N, Ohtsuka T, Tamura K, et al. Intraductal papillary mucinous neoplasms of the pancreas with distinct pancreatic ductal adenocarcinomas are frequently of gastric subtype. Ann Surg. 2013;258:141–51.

Ingkakul T, Sadakari Y, Ienaga J, et al. Predictors of the presence of concomitant invasive ductal carcinoma in intraductal papillary mucinous neoplasm of the pancreas. Ann Surg. 2010;251:70–5.

Japan Pancreas Society. Classification of pancreatic carcinoma. 3rd ed. Tokyo: Kanehara; 2011.
Kobayashi G, Fujita N, Noda Y, et al. Lateral spread along the main pancreatic duct in branch-duct intraductal papillary-mucinous neoplasms of the pancreas: usefulness of intraductal ultrasonography for its evaluation. Dig Endosc. 2011;23:62–8.
Maguchi H, Tanno S, Mizuno N, et al. Natural history of branch duct intraductal papillary mucinous neoplasms of the pancreas: a multicenter study in Japan. Pancreas. 2011;40:364–70.
Matthaei H, Norris AL, Tsiatis AC, et al. Clinicopathological characteristics and molecular analyses of multifocal intraductal papillary mucinous neoplasms of the pancreas. Ann Surg. 2012;255:326–33.
Mino-Kenudson M, Fernández-del Castillo C, Baba Y, et al. Prognosis of invasive intraductal papillary mucinous neoplasm depends on histological and precursor epithelial subtypes. Gut. 2011;60:1712–20.
Mori Y, Ohtsuka T, Kono H, et al. Management strategy for multifocal branch duct intraductal papillary mucinous neoplasms of the pancreas. Pancreas. 2012;41:1008–12.
Ohtsuka T, Kono H, Tanabe R, et al. Follow-up study after resection of intraductal papillary mucinous neoplasm of the pancreas; special references to the multifocal lesions and development of ductal carcinoma in the remnant pancreas. Am J Surg. 2012;204:44–8.
Ohtsuka T, Ideno N, Aso T, et al. Role of endoscopic retrograde pancreatography to detect early pancreatic ductal carcinoma concomitant with intraductal papillary mucinous neoplasm of the pancreas. J Hepatobiliary Pancreat Sci. 2013;20:356–61.
Okada K, Imaizumi T, Hirabayashi K, et al. The distance of the tumor spread in the main pancreatic duct of an intraductal papillary-mucinous neoplasm: where to resect and how to predict it. J Hepatobiliary Pancreat Sci. 2010;17:516–22.
Partelli S, Fernández-del Castillo C, Bassi C, et al. Invasive intraductal papillary mucinous carcinomas of the pancreas. Predictors of survival and the role of lymph node ratio. Ann Surg. 2010;251:477–82.
Poultsides GA, Reddy S, Cameron JL, et al. Histopathologic basis for the favorable survival after resection of intraductal papillary mucinous neoplasm-associated invasive adenocarcinoma of the pancreas. Ann Surg. 2010;251:470–6.
Reid-Lombardo KM, Mathis KL, Wood CM, et al. Frequency of extrapancreatic neoplasms in intraductal papillary mucinous neoplasm of the pancreas. Implication for management. Ann Surg. 2010;251:64–9.
Rodriguez JR, Salvia R, Crippa S, et al. Branch-duct intraductal papillary mucinous neoplasms: observations in 145 patients who underwent resection. Gastroenterology. 2007;133:72–9.
Sadakari Y, Ohuchida K, Nakata K, et al. Invasive carcinoma derived from non-intestinal type intraductal papillary mucinous neoplasm of the pancreas has a poorer prognosis than that derived from intestinal type. Surgery. 2010;147:812–7.
Salvia R, Fernández-del Castillo C, Bassi C, et al. Main-duct intraductal papillary mucinous neoplasms of the pancreas. Clinical predictors of malignancy and long-term survival following resection. Ann Surg. 2004;239:678–87.
Sawai Y, Yamao K, Bhatia V, et al. Development of pancreatic cancers during long-term follow-up of side-branch intraductal papillary mucinous neoplasms. Endoscopy. 2010;42:1077–84.
Sohn TA, Yeo CJ, Cameron JL, et al. Intraductal papillary mucinous neoplasms of the pancreas. An updated experience. Ann Surg. 2004;239:788–99.
Sugiyama M, Atomi Y. Extrapancreatic neoplasms occur with unusual frequency in patients with intraductal papillary mucinous tumors of the pancreas. Am J Gastroenterol. 1999;94:470–3.
Tada M, Kawabe T, Arizumi M, et al. Pancreatic cancer in patients with pancreatic cystic lesions: a prospective study in 197 patients. Clin Gastroenterol Hepatol. 2006;4:1265–70.
Tanaka M, Fernández-del Castillo C, Adsay V, et al. International consensus guidelines 2012 for the management of IPMN and MCN of the pancreas. Pancreatology. 2012;12:183–97.
Tanno S, Nakano Y, Koizumi K, et al. Pancreatic ductal adenocarcinomas in long-term follow-up patients with branch duct intraductal papillary mucinous neoplasms. Pancreas. 2010a;39:36–40.
Tanno S, Nakano Y, Sugiyama Y, et al. Incidence of synchronous and metachronous pancreatic carcinoma in 168 patients with branch duct intraductal papillary mucinous neoplasms. Pancreatology. 2010b;10:173–8.

Uehara H, Nakaizumi A, Ishikawa O, et al. Development of ductal carcinoma of the pancreas during follow-up of branch duct intraductal papillary mucinous neoplasms of the pancreas. Gut. 2008;57:1561–5.

Wada K, Kozarek RA, Traverso LW. Outcomes following resection of invasive and noninvasive intraductal papillary mucinous neoplasms of the pancreas. Am J Surg. 2005;189:632–7.

White R, D'Angelica M, Katabi N, et al. Fate of the remnant pancreas after resection of noninvasive intraductal papillary mucinous neoplasm. J Am Coll Surg. 2007;204:987–95.

Yamaguchi K, Ohuchida J, Ohtsuka T, et al. Intraductal papillary-mucinous tumor of the pancreas concomitant with ductal carcinoma of the pancreas. Pancreatology. 2002;2:484–90.

Yamaguchi K, Kanemitsu S, Hatori T, et al. Pancreatic ductal adenocarcinoma derived from IPMN and pancreatic ductal adenocarcinoma concomitant with IPMN. Pancreas. 2011;40:571–80.

Yopp AC, Katabi N, Janakos M, et al. Invasive carcinoma arising in intraductal papillary mucinous neoplasms of the pancreas. A match control study with conventional pancreatic ductal adenocarcinoma. Ann Surg. 2011;253:968–74.

Index

M. Tanaka (ed.), *Intraductal Papillary Mucinous Neoplasm of the Pancreas*,
DOI 10.1007/978-4-431-54472-2, © Springer Japan 2014

MIX
Papier aus verantwortungsvollen Quellen
Paper from responsible sources
FSC® C105338

If you have any concerns about our products,
you can contact us on
ProductSafety@springernature.com

In case Publisher is established outside the EU,
the EU authorized representative is:
Springer Nature Customer Service Center GmbH
Europaplatz 3, 69115 Heidelberg, Germany

Printed by Libri Plureos GmbH
in Hamburg, Germany